Health Promotion ....:

Strategies for Reaching
Diverse Populations
at the Workplace

Stephen Ramirez, MPH

a publication of the Wellness Councils of America

Wellness Councils of America is a national nonprofit
organization dedicated to promoting healthier lifestyles
for all Americans, especially through
health promotion activities at the worksite.

This project was produced with funding, in part, from

The JM Foundation
Metropolitan Life Foundation
The Prudential Foundation
CIGNA Foundation
AT&T Foundation
Union Pacific Railroad

ISBN 0-9628334-3-6

CREDITS:

Editor: Sandra Wendel, Wellness Councils of America

Design: Freestyle Graphics, Omaha

LA Design, Omaha

Cover: SuperStock. Artist, Diana Ong, a multimedia specialist, originally created the cover art, entitled *Crowd IV*, in watercolor. She attended the National Academy of Fine Arts and the School of Visual Arts in New York.

Wellness Councils of America
Community Health Plaza, Suite 311
7101 Newport Ave.
Omaha, NE 68152-2175
(402) 572-3590

Acknowledgments

Contributions to the development of this book have been made by a number of knowledgeable and respected medical, health promotion, and education professionals. Of particular note is the contribution made by the staff of The American Institute for Managing Diversity—one of the pioneers and trail blazers in helping corporate America manage diversity. Many of the Institute's concepts, ideas, and perspectives helped shape the sections of this book that define diversity and managing diversity in worksite health promotion. Specifically, thanks to Cleveland Clarke, Maureen Hunter, and Michael S. Jacobson, MD.

Additional significant contributions have been made by a blue-ribbon panel of reviewers. Their critique, comments, and insights in reviewing the draft manuscript were extremely helpful in shaping the final publication. My sincere thanks to the following:

Susan Burke, MEd
Manager, Health and Fitness
Xerox Corp. (Calif.)

Moon S. Chen, PhD, MPH
Professor
Dept. of Preventive Medicine
The Ohio State University
Editor, *Asian American and Pacific Islander Journal of Health*

Carolee Dodge-Francis
Executive Director
Wellness Council of the Upper Peninsula in Michigan

Ashley Files
Coordinator, Community-based and Worksite Health Promotion Projects
Office of Disease Prevention and Health Promotion

Agnes K. Hernandez
Development Director
National Kidney Foundation of Nebraska
former Community Relations Director, American Diabetes
  Association (Northern Illinois affiliate)

Brick Lancaster, MA, CHES
Assoc. Director for Health Education Practice and Policy
Division of Chronic Disease Control and Community Intervention
Centers for Disease Control and Prevention

Joe Leutzinger, PhD
Manager, Health Promotion
Union Pacific Railroad

Eileen J. Lourie, MD
Phoenix Area Indian Health Service

Henry Montes, MPH
Asst. Director, Minority Health
Centers for Disease Control and Prevention

Michael O'Donnell, MBA, MPH
Publisher
American Journal of Health Promotion

Amelie G. Ramirez, DrPH, MPH, CHES
Assoc. Director, South Texas Health Research Center
Assoc. Professor of Family Practice

David Steurer
Executive Director
Wellness Council of West Virginia

Craig Washington, EdD
Chair, Science and Applied Technologies Division
Northern Virginia Community College

I also wish to thank Dr. Harold Davis for his thoughtful and well-crafted foreword. Dr. Davis has been a pioneer and early advocate of the diversity and health promotion concepts in corporate America.

When this project was on the drawing board, health promotion planners in the nationwide network of the Wellness Councils of America were asked to help shape this book. I thank them for their early input.

It should also be noted that this book would not have been possible without the total commitment and support of the staff of the Wellness Councils of America. This organization is defining the important and emerging issues for corporate wellness programs. I specifically thank Sandra Wendel, director of communication, who passionately pursued this project for years and made it happen, and to Harold Kahler, WELCOA's president, for giving me this opportunity to make a contribution.

Sincere thanks go to Kelley Juhrend for organizing and typing the initial drafts. Her contribution is integral to the completed document.

Many of the processes and principles described in this book have been implemented in Fresno County with the support and encouragement of the Health Services Agency administration. I want to acknowledge and thank George Bleth and Gary Carozza for their support.

Special recognition and gratitude is also to be accorded to Arthur L. Williams, Jr., director of training, Boys and Girls Clubs of America, Southeast Region. His guidance, mentorship, knowledge, and experience in assessment, evaluation, and human resources management was of tremendous value to me.

Finally, and most important, I dedicate this book to my parents. Many of the beliefs, values, and practices they instilled in me have resulted in numerous professional successes and achievements—including the writing of this book. My parents continue to teach me more about the concepts and importance of recognizing diversity than this book can adequately portray. My completion of this book is written testimony to their parenting and the love and respect I have for them.

Stephen Ramirez, MPH
Fresno, Calif.

Contents

Foreword

Harold M. Davis, MD
Vice President—Human Resources
Employee Health Service, Managing Diversity, and Corporate Training and Development
The Prudential

The year 2000 is rapidly approaching with its impending demographic, sociocultural, and political shifts. Our nation will be moving from a society that has historically been shaped to meet the needs of a dominant group, to one where the diversity of its citizens will determine how our institutions function. The viability of the nation demands a shift to inclusion for those who have been excluded.

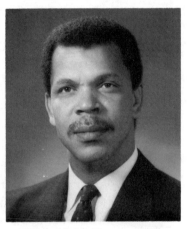

Harold M. Davis, MD

While America has taken its first steps to address the oncoming tide of social change with a proliferation of initiatives to meet the demands of the diversity wave, the question remains: Have we in the health professions begun to make ourselves, our services, and our institutions relevant to a diverse constituency? If current models of health education, delivery systems, and health profiles of Americans are indicators of things to come, the answer would have to be "no."

Our present health model assumes, wrongly, that common ideals and goals regarding health motivate all Americans in the same way and to the same degree. This has resulted in a one-size-fits-all health system, which has dominated the philosophy and structure of American medicine. This assumption, and the systems that result from that assumption, however, negate the concept of diversity and, in turn, exclude those who are in desperate need of health care because they cannot align themselves to the current health care structure.

If we are to successfully meet the health needs of all we serve, we must agree that our current health models (the system itself and our health views) will not get us to where we need to be. Success lies before us, but it will only be achieved when our health systems and providers are able to function amid diversity. This diversity will have to include differences in "health status," which may be significantly affected by race, gender, social class, culture, and physical ability, among others, as well as by diversity in "health views" among our employees as to what is health and how to attain it.

It is also imperative that we approach the transformation of American medicine with a strong sense of urgency. For while we debate whether or not there is a health crisis in the nation, Americans are dying now!

These are needless deaths. They challenge the efficiency of our health system and seriously question the humanity of the American people. A disturbing part of our nation's history, and its current health report card, is the unacceptably high and shamefully excessive death rates that are flagrantly evident for large segments of the American population—in particular, for African Americans, Hispanics/Latinos, Native Americans, and Asian and Pacific Islanders.

Excessive death rates have gone unnoticed by large segments of our health care establishment and, alarmingly, persist despite tremendous gains made in medical science, technology, and numbers of personnel committed to the health professions.

As you will learn through this important book by Steve Ramirez, 80 percent of the excess deaths experienced by America's racial and ethnic populations are caused by (1) cancer, (2) cardiovascular disease and stroke, (3) infant mortality and low birth weight, (4) chemical dependency, particularly alcoholism and IV drug use, (5) homicide, with suicide and intentional injuries contributing significant numbers, and (6) diabetes. To this list we must now add AIDS, caused by an epidemic of HIV infection in African American and Hispanic communities.

Health education and outreach programs for diverse groups—among them a disproportionate number of racial and ethnic populations—to address these unhealthy outcomes are not readily available. The sad truth is that the wellness movement in America has not recruited diverse groups to its ranks and has been characterized by them as elitist.

For members of many racial and ethnic groups, wellness, as currently defined, is far beyond their reach. They cannot afford health club memberships, high-priced fitness gear, or "designer" health foods. They are doing all they can to house and clothe themselves and just plain eat! The wellness movement has to come down to earth where the common man, woman, and child are if it ever hopes to be a relevant force in their lives.

Culturally competent and specific action plans to address the health needs of diverse populations are noticeably missing from our nation's health care system. Also, when marginal attempts are made to address their health problems and needs, there is frequently a "blame the victim" defense mounted by health care institutions when their outreach efforts have not yielded the desired results. The victims are blamed for (1) not appreciating what is done for them, (2) not using what is provided, and (3) continuing to practice lifestyles that perpetuate high rates of morbidity and mortality.

In defense of the so-called victims, you should remember that preventive medicine, such as lifestyle enhancement and appropriate use of the health system, is a hard sell even for those who have the resources to address today's health needs and also plan for a better tomorrow. It is a particularly difficult sell for those who are concerned primarily with staying alive today, let alone tomorrow. We, as health care professionals, need user-friendly programs and outreach initiatives; we must also consider their life circumstances and options in our health promotion planning.

The issues in this book should be of immediate concern to you as you plan your health promotion programming. The American health care system is being pressed into relevant interaction with its constituents. You, as providers of health promotion services, are also being challenged to provide meaningful, cost-beneficial service for your employees. To neglect the needs of diverse groups of employees challenges the relevance and value of your program. Meeting the medical needs of racial and ethnic groups and others in your organization may represent the greatest medical benefits cost-saving opportunity available to you.

A chain is made stronger by strengthening the weakest links, and, for now, the weakest link is the state of health for many racial and ethnic populations and other diverse groups in America.

Additional benefits may also result when your health messages and lifestyle recommendations are transferred to family members. You truly can create the opportunity to influence their health status as well. When you use culturally sensitive health messages to train employees about the health care system and teach them to be better health care consumers, and when you help them make healthy lifestyle choices and motivate them to succeed, what better way to help employees change their health profiles?

Developing cultural competency in our health care delivery system and personnel is, admittedly, a challenge. It is not, however, beyond our capacity. To succeed, we will need to care to a higher degree, be willing to adapt to a changing social order, have a broader sense of constituency, own the task before us, and be patient and steadfast in our conviction that meeting the needs of all our clients "MATTERS" to us.

Let me offer a formula. Here's how you can demonstrate that reaching your diverse employee groups matters:

M arket — with culturally sensitive material

A ccess — made easier for the user

T raining — staff about diversity in all its dimensions including cultural, racial, and ethnic differences

T reatment — of different populations

E ducation — of your clients in a respectful way

R esearch — on what works

S olutions — that work should be supported

Read on, so we all can achieve "health promotion for all."

Introduction

Cleveland Clarke, Jr.
Director, Marketing and Development
The American Institute for Managing Diversity, Inc.
Atlanta

The management of diversity within the context of health promotion—the topic of this book—has reached a critical level of national attention. Every organization, whether public or private, governmental, educational, or nonprofit, must, if they are not already doing so, address diversity.

Old and "unconscious prescriptions for success"—which influence our thinking regarding how to treat patients, what types of health programs should a company offer its employees, what systems or policies should be written that will govern how resources should be allocated, and spell out the roles and levels of responsibilities of management and employees—must undergo a new level of professional scrutiny. We may discover that what worked in the past may or may not be relevant today. The simple fact is that our internal and external environment has changed and continues to change.

The process of examining these "unconscious prescriptions for success" is the first step in understanding the drivers within a given organization's culture. Ultimately, we want to reach a point where we are able to ensure that the culture of any organization is sufficiently capable of responding to the health needs of its employees. The stakes are high, and there are no short cuts.

In this book, Steve Ramirez offers a new way of thinking about health promotion that has important implications for today's generation and future generations. His thoughtful reflections on this topic make his findings both timely and a meaningful collection of writings for serious-minded health promotion professionals.

Steve incorporates the notion of the three E's in his very own success formula: education, economics, and the environment. He looks at each from an organizational context. If these concepts are successfully applied, Steve believes an organization will be able to create an internal environment that naturally promotes the health and well-being of its employees.

A synergistic approach to health management is not only smart but essential. In fact, The American Institute for Managing Diversity, Inc., defines diversity as the collective mixture of similarities and differences within a diverse context. Whether that diverse context is functional, geographic, global, based on lifestyles, related to race or gender, or measured in some other way, you—the practitioner—must consider each dimension as you develop your health promotion strategies.

We commend Steve's practical advice to you as you launch your health promotion efforts. We hope they will help you in your journey.

1

Defining Diversity in Workplace Health Promotion

The Dimensions of Diversity

Your first task is to identify the various groups in your workforce, understand their needs, and design programs and services accordingly. You may have to expand the breadth of program offerings beyond those that, in past years, served a particular employee profile. Some wellness programs evolved from "executives-only" saunas and showers or didn't include women or blue-collar employees in the plant.

The dimensions that need to be taken into consideration include—but are not limited to—health risks associated with the following:

- race
- ethnicity
- culture and level of acculturation
- gender
- educational levels
- access to resources
- physical challenges

Written with contributions from Maureen Hunter, Director of Education, The American Institute for Managing Diversity, Inc.

- lifestyle
- geographical location and background
- sexual orientation
- work schedule
- marital status
- language spoken
- occupation
- economic status
- age or generation
- family structure and support system

At first blush, designing programs to meet the needs of such dissimilar constituents may seem daunting and complex. But the benefits of serving one group may spill over and serve others as well. Therefore, this book looks, not at every possible difference, but at the larger differences among employees and their health risks.

Accordingly, this book concentrates on the major dimensions of diversity—race, ethnicity, and culture. These dimensions encompass populations or groups— based on a review of their health status, needs, and interests—who will require a more targeted or tailored approach in your worksite health promotion delivery system.

You will find out information concerning the continuing and persistent health and disease problems facing the country's four main racial and ethnic populations: African Americans, Asian and Pacific Islanders, Hispanics (Latinos), and Native Americans. Many of these racial and ethnic groups continue to experience disproportionately higher rates of disability and death related to chronic and communicable disease.

Wellness: Health Care Reform That Works

This book links the concepts of health and diversity—perhaps for the first time for many health promotion professionals and health planners in worksites across the country. Far too often, both issues are thought of as **costs** associated with the organization's employee population rather than as factors that **contribute,** significantly, to the organization's effectiveness, bottom line, and long-term viability.

An investment in health promotion and in managing diversity pays off in the contributions made by a workforce that's highly productive, that uses every employee's talents fully, and that shares a commitment to achieving the organization's mission and objectives. *Managing diversity* is defined by The American Institute for Managing Diversity as the process of enabling, empowering, and influencing, not in the sense of controlling or manipulation.

By linking diversity with workplace health promotion, a company embraces the notion of creating a work environment that heightens the potential for all employees (empowers) to be productive, to be healthy, and to contribute to the company.

For the business leaders, small business owners, corporate managers, or administrators who are not yet convinced of the methods or philosophy of managing diversity, consider this: Your competitors are already or will soon be gaining significant advantages in their employee base as America's workforce continues to grow more diverse.

The same can be said about corporate health promotion. The concept has evolved from being simply an executive perk—or not existing at all—to a business practice in more than 81 percent of companies across the country, according to a 1992 government survey—because wellness offers business advantages with measurable payoffs. [1]

If your company is not managing for diversity or integrating health promotion into your corporate culture, your company may be at a distinct business **dis**advantage. There's no question—American business operates in a global marketplace where corporations, small businesses, and industries must learn to compete and be successful working with other countries and various cultures as well as competing with market forces at home.

To remain competitive in this global economy, America's businesses must capitalize on the abilities and skills a diverse workforce offers. Creating and sustaining a productive, healthy, and supportive work environment for all employees regardless of their background can lead to business success.

Look at the business side of the equation. Let's consider the health care costs to your company if you do not have a worksite health promotion program that actively involves all employee groups. Changes in how health care is delivered and paid for will only slightly affect the spiraling costs of health care itself. The real value for your health care dollar is in assuring that all employees participate in cost-reducing health promotion and prevention programs at your workplace.

"For small business owners who often measure profits in thousands—not millions—of dollars, the net effect of an employee wellness program could mean the difference between profit and loss," according to William M. Kizer, chairman of Central States Health & Life Co. of Omaha and founding chairman of the Wellness Councils of America.

Organizations that value, recognize, and support diversity in the worksite can motivate employees to be more productive, to make healthy lifestyle choices, and to contribute to the quality of life in their own community. But only those businesses that actively put the philosophy of managing diversity to work for better quality, services, and employees will gain a competitive advantage and create a work environment that is truly health promoting for all.

Diversity. What Is It?

Diversity. When you read this term, what images are displayed in your mind? How do you define this term in your workplace health promotion program? What does it mean to you personally? Perhaps it sounds like just another politically correct buzzword that will evolve into some other euphemism next year. Whatever you call it, let's discuss the meaning behind the word.

Pacific Gas & Electric defines diversity as "any difference in race, gender, age, language, physical characteristics, disabilities, sexual orientation, economic status, parental status, education, geographic origin, profession, lifestyle, religion, or position in the hierarchy of the organization." PG&E's view on managing diversity "requires the creation of an open, supportive, responsive organization in which differences are understood, encouraged, appreciated, and managed."

R. Roosevelt Thomas, Jr., president and founder of The American Institute for Managing Diversity defines diversity to include—quite simply—"everyone. . . . In this expanded context, white males are as diverse as their colleagues. A commitment to diversity is a commitment to all employees, not an attempt at preferential treatment." [2]

To expand Roosevelt Thomas's definition to include workplace health promotion: Diversity incorporates a complete examination of the health needs, interests, and issues of all employees. Particular attention and concern should be given to any employee group that, through an objective data analysis, can be considered high risk or at risk for specific health problems, diseases, and disability.

America has always been and continues to be a nation of diversity—not only diversity of race, ethnicity, and gender but differences of educational level, personality, skills, thought, physical abilities, interests, and other categories between and among individuals and groups of people. Where did we **ever** get the notion that all whites, Hispanics (Latinos), African Americans, Asian and Pacific Islanders, Native Americans, European Americans, Italians, Irish, women, Texans, New Yorkers, artists, technicians, high school graduates, college professors—you get the idea— always think and act in categorically similar fashion?

Have the media, history books, and marketing campaigns limited our ability to consider each and every human being as a unique individual regardless of his or her race, ethnicity, or gender?

To be truly effective in addressing diversity issues as part of health promotion, you must make it clear that your program is not limited to one or a few specific groups of employees. Just as you want to offer more than a running club for a few serious marathoners, more than aerobic exercise for the office staff, more than nutrition classes for the overweight, more than smoking cessation for the smokers—you want to include programs to meet the needs of your entire workforce.

You must take the approach that diversity exists for everyone, and the strategies you use can be tailored for both individual and group needs as they are identified. Your program can include activities for both homogeneous (similar) and heterogenous (different) groups of employees. Recognize that these groups tend to be self-selected. In other words, people who want to walk during lunch will tend to do so as a group; smokers cluster around the outdoor smoking areas and form friendships based on their habits; tennis players set times to meet at local courts.

Majority, Not Minority

We have chosen to avoid the term *minority* in this book because, in the United States, four major racial and ethnic groups constitute the majority in more than 2,000 counties, cities, towns, and other places, according to the Census Bureau.

Members of these four racial and ethnic populations compose the majority in six of the eight American cities with more than 1 million people: New York, Los Angeles, Chicago, Houston, Detroit, and Dallas. [3]

More than 43 percent of California's population is composed of the following groups: 25.8 percent Hispanic; 9.6 percent Asian and Pacific Islander Americans; 7.4 percent African American; and 0.8 percent Native American (from 1990 Census). These groups—hardly characterized as minorities—make up 40 percent of California's workforce, up from 30 percent in 1980, according to the state Department of Finance.

In 51 of the USA's largest cities (population at least 100,000), African Americans, Hispanics, Asian and Pacific Islander Americans, and Native Americans collectively are more than half the population: for example, East Los Angeles, 97.2 percent; Miami, 87.8 percent; Atlanta, 69.7 percent. [4]

One size does not fit all. Workplace health planners should take a marketing approach and tailor the programs to the individual needs of the customer—in this case, the customer is the employee.

Building relationships with employees where they feel valued, respected, and included in your health promotion program will be a challenging task. You don't have the ability to influence every area. However, acknowledging in your program that each employee brings a unique set of characteristics, needs, interests, concerns, and problems to the worksite—and demonstrating honesty and thoughtfulness in your approach to them—should create opportunities for you to earn the trust and respect of diverse groups of people.

A Nation of Immigrants

America has always been a nation of immigrants and has gained considerable strength, wisdom, and knowledge from the achievements and contributions of diverse racial, ethnic, and cultural populations.

Cultural diversity, multicultural, bicultural—these terms have received increasing attention over the last decade. America has historically been a nation of diversity beginning with the civilizations that existed on this continent prior to the arrival of people from other continents, and that pattern continues today.

Take a moment to consider the diversity of your own family background. Where did your parents and grandparents originate? Another country? A different city or state? Perhaps your great grandfather entered this country though Ellis Island, or walked across the Rio Grande, or landed at LAX. Perhaps your ancestors can be traced to the *Mayflower*, or maybe your relatives greeted the *Mayflower* on its arrival at Plymouth Rock. All of these issues and more contribute to your individual diversity—how you view the world and your beliefs and values.

To incorporate diversity into workplace health promotion, you must examine your own diversity first. Then look at the diversity of your workforce.

You can't grab a standardized, ready-to-use package of health promotion programs and materials off the shelf and address all the needs of your workforce. The processes, guidelines, resources, and examples provided in this book are presented in a manner for you to move away from any preexisting beliefs or attitudes you may currently have in regard to the health needs, interests, and practices of any group employed at your worksite. The processes outlined here will move you toward a complete, honest, accurate, and objective analysis of program development in cooperation with representatives of diverse groups of employees.

It is imperative that you place yourself in a learning and awareness mode as you examine the health and medical research and data that have been gathered on specific racial and ethnic groups as well as consider individually their health needs and interests through your own process at the worksite. You will learn how to use a balance of empirical, anecdotal, and experiential information derived from your employee groups to help you achieve a health promotion program that addresses the diversity of your workforce.

You are provided with ideas, information, and examples that may apply to your particular worksite and workforce. Community-based health promotion programs have had some success using many of the approaches described in this book. However, worksites have not moved as quickly to approach these areas in the same manner as many public health and community-based organizations have done. Therefore, successful examples in the workplace are hard to find.

A "Labor" Issue

One of the most significant hotel industry labor force issues is the high turnover of the workforce. At the Irvine Marriott in Orange County, California, where more than 80 percent of employees are Hispanic (36% are Spanish speaking), turnover among female housekeepers was unusually high when the women had children. Many quit and never returned to the workforce.

The hotel hoped to encourage them to return to work—and many wanted to return to work—after maternity leave. The problem was that, generally, staff were not aware of their benefits. At the same time, the hotel management wanted to provide educational information on child-care choices and prenatal care issues.

Calling on community health practitioners and the Public Health Service, the hotel staged a workshop called "How to Be a Working Mother" and geared it toward expectant and working mothers—and conducted much in Spanish.

"If we do good things, that information will spread into the Latino community," said John Masamori, the hotel's director of human resources. "Unless we offer something a little special, we don't have a workforce."

Coming to Terms: A Perspective on Race, Ethnicity, and Culture

It is important for you, as you read this book, to review the concepts of race, ethnicity, and culture as these are defined by the individual employees you serve. Rather than looking at your workforce and asking: *Who are they?* Ask: *How do they identify themselves?*

Individuals must be viewed as portraits of diversity—mixtures of different demographics and values. For example, consider the various health promotion needs of these employees:

- The single, young African American male
- The middle-aged, divorced, highly educated white male whose children live out of state
- Two newly arrived immigrants from Southeast Asia: one a highly educated professional, the other with few years of formal schooling in his native country; neither speak English; both enter the labor force in jobs that provide no health insurance
- A young, married, American Indian construction worker living in an urban area
- The young, single-parent Puerto Rican female
- The young, single-parent white female

These examples are not intended to portray stereotypes but to remind us of the dimensions of diversity and just how disparate the workforce has become. [5]

In March 1993, the Centers for Disease Control and Prevention and the Agency for Toxic Substances and Disease Registry conducted a workshop to promote discussions on issues of race and ethnicity in public health data collection.[6] Participants in the workshops agreed on a number of general principles:

1. The **concepts of race and ethnicity are not well defined or consistently measured** [our emphasis] among federal agencies. Common concepts and measures are essential for effective public health surveillance.

2. The concept of race as assessed in public health surveillance is a social measure. Biological or genetic reference, or both, should be made with **extreme caution** [our emphasis]. The relationship between concepts of race and ethnicity should be clarified.

3. Effective use of race and ethnicity in public health surveillance rests on an **understanding of the socioeconomic and cultural factors that underlie differences in health status** [our emphasis]. Racial and ethnic information should be supplemented with relevant information on socioeconomic and cultural variables [discussed in this book in chapter 2].

4. Public health information on racial and ethnic populations can be used to stigmatize populations and reinforce traditional stereotypes. Therefore, when race and ethnic information is collected, it is essential to explain why the information is collected, how it is determined, and what it means. [The sample employee survey in the appendix may help you discover the answers to how employees define themselves and their racial, ethnic, and cultural backgrounds.]

5. To collect valid and reliable surveillance data, it is essential to assess the meaning and use of concepts of race, ethnicity, ancestry, and national origin among the different segments of the U.S. population.

6. It is essential that the racial and ethnic populations that are being surveyed participate in the planning and overall design of public health surveillance programs and in prevention, intervention, and evaluation activities directed toward improving their health status [use the techniques discussed in chapter 3 in forming your employee advisory committee for your health promotion program planning].

In addition to these general principles, workshop participants made the following recommendations, among others:

■ Valid and reliable concepts of race, ethnicity, and related notions, such as ancestry or national origin, should be explored. The interrelations among these concepts should also be investigated. It may be, for example, that what is measured as "race" in public health surveillance is closer to the concept of "ethnicity" (that is, self-perceived memberships in populations defined by diverse criteria, including common ancestry, nationality, culture, language, and physical appearance).

■ Social, economic, and political forces underlying differences in health status among racial and ethnic populations should be investigated and reported in population studies of health status.

■ To assure valid and reliable responses to surveillance questions such as "What is your race?" and "What is your ancestry?" it is important to assess concepts of and language for race, ancestry, ethnicity, and related notions among diverse segments of the U.S. population. [7]

This book is not intended as a defining document or authority on the subjects of race, ethnicity, or culture as these terms relate to diversity and worksite health promotion. But it is evident from the CDC workshop information that these terms and issues are under considerable national discussion and in essence are a "work in progress."

Use this book, then, as a starting point on your marathon as you reach out to serve diverse groups of employees. This process is indeed a marathon, not a sprint, and you must make a considerable effort to examine issues, topics, definitions, and terms that may be uncomfortable to some; difficult to negotiate; and, at times, controversial.

Your task is to develop an appropriate way to gather racial, ethnic, cultural, socioeconomic, and other categories of information from the employees you are serving in your health promotion program. The key element in this process is to allow employees the opportunity to define themselves, their diversity, and their group affiliations as they believe appropriate.

Developing a Successful Formula— Education, Economics, Environment

No single strategy or approach works for all businesses attempting to manage diversity in the organization and within the health promotion program. Each company must make a commitment to carefully examine this issue with management and employee groups and devote time, effort, and, where needed, the resources (financial and people) to make management of diversity a success.

Start with a mission statement to guide your health promotion program. This simple but powerful statement becomes the roadmap for you and your employee advisory group (and we'll discuss the importance and makeup of this group in chapter 3). Here's one example, adapted and used with permission from SC Johnson Wax in Racine, Wis., a member of the Wisconsin Wellness Council:

> MISSION: **Our workforce will reflect diversity at all levels, seek and value differences of opinion and views, be flexible in accommodating work/ family issues, and develop the talents of all people in order to improve our creativity, productivity, and competitiveness. Our health promotion program will encourage people to take responsibility for their own health and to make wellness a way of living a longer, healthier life.**

? *"My worksite does not employ large numbers of workers. Do I still need to conduct this major process to achieve diversity management in my health promotion programs?"*

Yes and no. A lot of it depends on what you find out during your employee needs and interests survey. No matter the size of the organization, all worksites should have developed an environment which recognizes, supports, and reinforces diversity as it relates to productivity and health status of employees.

Don't cut corners. Yes, many of us would like the "quick and dirty" method of developing and implementing program activities. However, think of it this way: Would you want the construction company building your new home to spend more or less time on the foundation? Would you prefer your mechanic to spend more or less time adjusting and fixing your car's brakes and steering system? Do you want your physician to spend more or less time analyzing and diagnosing a persistent medical problem for you or your children?

Consider these steps as you develop your own mission statement to link diversity and health promotion:

STEP 1—Identify the existing company corporate philosophy. It's the one that describes why the organization exists. Be guided by it as you develop a mission statement within the framework of your health promotion program.

STEP 2—Review with your employee advisory group (including executives and managers) how the current mission statement can be adapted to include issues of diversity and the health and well-being of employees.

STEP 3—Ask employees to submit a revised mission statement that's compatible with your company's overall mission and be sure to work through your employee advisory group. Submit suggestions to senior executives for input and approval.

What can you do in your health promotion program that will help you carry out your mission? Consider the three E's— education, economics, and environment—as you plan your strategies.

Education and Management of Diversity

Your strategies for developing and implementing any health promotion or other human resource program must consider the range of educational levels and abilities among employees. For some employees, English may be their second language, and a pamphlet on high blood pressure in Spanish, perhaps, may better fit their needs. Others may have difficulty reading and would prefer video presentations, for example.

Also, think about printing training manuals or benefits policies in more than one language, if the need exists, and perhaps at a more appropriate readability level. Acknowledge various cultural and ethnic celebrations such as El Cinco de Mayo and the Hmong New Year, or plan events to recognize all cultures and ethnic groups and their contributions. A potluck with traditional dishes is an excellent way to bring together employees who don't normally socialize with one another.

In any message, worksite health promotion planners will want to be culturally relevant. *Culturally relevant* can be defined in different ways. If you survey the needs and interests of employees, they will define for you what is culturally relevant. Let them tell you who they are and about their background and cultural belief system. Then you can create educational materials, events, and activities that incorporate the cultural images, art, music, foods, positive health values, beliefs, and practices of all groups represented at the worksite.

A Fundamental Commitment, Not Tokenism

"Worksite health promotion programs for ethnic/racial people cannot be isolated or compartmentalized. They have to be integrated into and integral to the ongoing worksite health promotion. To be effective, they have to be a natural outgrowth of a fundamental commitment to diversity that is embodied throughout the organization. This means that offering one session once a year on a topic of special relevance to African Americans or Latinos is useless tokenism because it does nothing to address those groups in an ongoing way, nor does it do anything to raise whites' awareness of the population," according to health promotion researchers Marilyn Aguirre-Molina and Carlos W. Molina.[8]

Remember, cultural relevance depends on the perception and attitudes of the people employed at your worksite. Do not expect to pick up a book or video to learn everything you need to know about any particular racial, cultural, or ethnic group. These resources are useful, but ultimately you must "personally" assess your employees through formal (written survey) and informal (focus groups, one-to-one) methods to truly learn what is culturally relevant, meaningful, or important to them and why.

Economics and Management of Diversity

Income and occupation of your employees will influence how you manage diversity in your health promotion program.

Consider these issues in planning your organization's educational program and in working with all employees: The needs of a single parent may be far different from the needs of the two-parent working family. For example, the single parent may simply not be able to attend health promotion classes outside the normal working hours because of child care commitments. The white-collar employees with support from an organized employee group may be more motivated to stop smoking than the blue-collar employees who might work long, tedious shifts through the night. And the type of industry you're in—manufacturing versus service—may influence employees' attitudes, abilities, and practices when it comes to health.

Companies that have successfully marketed products or services always factor in the economic equation when developing an advertising or sales campaign. You should do the same. Your goal is to get employees interested. You know you're successful if employees become involved and participate in your company-sponsored health promotion programs.

Environment and Management of Diversity

A company will achieve long-term success when it enhances (or creates) a business environment that values and recognizes the health and diversity of its employees. Employees' attitudes and behavior are shaped, reinforced, and perpetuated (negatively or positively) to a large degree by their work environment. This goes beyond the physical aspects of the workplace to include supervisor-employee relationships, company benefits and incentives, and promotional opportunities, among others.

At the heart of the philosophy of managing diversity is the belief that there are unconscious, underlying assumptions embedded in the fabric of the organization. Some of these assumptions about the culture may present the greatest impediment to the organization's ability to effectively manage diversity—and to create a healthful environment.

An example might help to illustrate this point:

> *Lee arrives early for work and leaves late. Lee's manager is constantly giving the employees in the department work to do after deciding how it should be done. The expectation is that once a task has been assigned, everything else will be put to the side until the "emergency" task is completed. Consequently, employees have a difficult time planning their work, because they are always being interrupted with an emergency assignment from the boss. Employees often miss or are late for breaks and lunch because of the demands of the work. Lee has suggestions on how the work could be accomplished more effectively and smoothly, but the boss has made it clear that Lee hasn't been around long enough to really understand how things are done. Lee's manager also expects employees to stay late, even if there is nothing in particular to do, because it is a sign of employee commitment and loyalty. Lee is diabetic and finds it difficult to maintain the eating schedule that will help keep blood sugar levels in check.*

From a managing diversity perspective, the organization's culture, as reflected in the manager's behavior, reinforces the notion that subordination is encouraged and that employees should work long hours to be a full member of the so-called family. Commitment to task and loyalty to one's boss is the measuring stick for excellence, in this example, even when doing so ignores the health needs of employees and their personal quality-of-life choices. All of these factors discourage the contributions that can be made by employees: new ideas and solutions, creativity, empowered participation, and being valued as a member of the organization where the work environment encourages or makes possible their fullest contribution.

From the perspective of promoting good health, the culture described at Lee's company creates stress and could, therefore, contribute to employees' health problems. And, for Lee, the uncertain break times and erratic lunch hours made managing diabetes through diet very difficult.

Corporate culture can, be powerful in shaping health promoting behaviors: Middle managers, for example, in a medium-sized insurance company might readily allow employees to take part in health promotion programs, but in the office across the street, managers think wellness is a waste of employees' time. The owner of the auto parts shop around the corner works night and day and expects employees to do the same, yet the partners in the downtown law firm recognize the benefits of encouraging employees to take regular vacations. The newspaper office designates no-smoking areas, yet the school district bans smoking completely. These examples reflect corporate culture—"the way things are around here"—either formally or informally, and they all affect employee attitudes, morale, productivity, and health.

Your job, as worksite health promotion planner, is to look at the corporate culture. You will find out how the values, norms, peer support, organizational support, underlying assumptions for success, and work climate affect employees and contribute to a healthy—or unhealthy—work environment.

Your goal, then, is to create an organizational culture that effectively supports the management of diversity and promotes health and wellness.

Measuring Your Success

You will want to look at your corporate culture—formally through an evaluation process and informally by simply looking at the outcomes. Informally, for example, assess how your company is meeting the needs of diverse employees from the perspective of affirmative action (AA), understanding differences (UD), or managing diversity (MD) and valuing differences (VD) through some of the following activities:

- Mentors and mentoring programs (AA or UD)
- A recruitment program that actively seeks diverse candidates (AA)
- Informational forums or awareness programs about different cultural groups in the workplace and/or community; social events with multicultural themes; monthly programs featuring a particular culture (UD)
- Teams and task forces that come from a variety of disciplines, levels, and cultural groups in the organization, including the all-volunteer employee advisory committee for health promotion (AA, UD, or MD)
- Educational and training interventions in how to work cooperatively with people with differences and similarities (MD)
- Educational and training interventions in how to communicate and work with people with differences and similarities (MD)
- In-house publications and other media that represent the diversity within the organization (UD)
- Advertising and other public media that reflect both the diversity within the company as well as within the marketplace or clientele served by the organization (AA)

- Orientation programs with an emphasis on diversity, such as acculturation for immigrant workers or overseas managers in how to work in a U.S. business environment (AA or UD)
- Programs that address the special needs of employees, not only in health promotion but in areas such as child care and elder care programs; legal services especially with immigration issues; literacy programs to help those employees who might have attended poorer schools or received inadequate training; relocation; and courses teaching English as a second language (MD)
- Valuing differences as an essential part of management development (VD)

Striking a Balance

This book does not offer solutions to every challenge you may face in your worksite program. However, it provides a perspective and process through which you can address the health needs and interests of everyone in your workforce. Throughout these chapters, you will find answers to many of the most-asked questions posed by health planners like yourself.

If you develop a workplan, as outlined in chapter 3, to include diversity and follow the processes suggested in this book, you will open new doors, create additional opportunities, and reach employees who have not yet participated in your health promotion programs. Sometimes they are called the "hard-to-reach" segment of the workforce. But these people are not necessarily hard to reach; they are perhaps not yet being reached, and that's your challenge. They haven't participated for a number of important reasons, and you'll find out about those barriers and how to overcome them.

If you are an experienced and time-tested "veteran" of worksite programs, then perhaps this book can serve as a means for you to revisit and rethink programs and services related to your employee groups. Use the suggested employee survey as part of your assessment process and peruse the tips on program evaluation. But, for most, the invaluable parts of this book lie in the program ideas and resources and in how to design educational materials for diverse populations within your workforce.

Those groups and their health risks are not always easily defined. We have decided to focus on a smaller range of diversity dimensions, that is, racial and ethnic diversity. It is important to note that other dimensions of diversity, mentioned earlier, are equally important and deserve the same level of careful and critical examination.

What follows is a discussion of the four main racial and ethnic populations. You will find out information in the next chapter concerning the continuing and persistent health and disease problems facing African Americans, Asian and Pacific Islander Americans, Hispanics (Latinos), and Native Americans. Members of these racial and ethnic groups continue to experience disproportionately higher rates of disability and death related to chronic and communicable disease.

To be truly effective, workplace health promotion programs must be tailored to address their health needs and interests, while serving the health needs of every employee.

24

? *"If diversity management is the concept we must embrace to insure all employees are served, why would we need to develop so-called separate programs for racial or ethnic populations?"*

If your "diversity" program model is effectively reaching these groups, then perhaps there is no need to consider this approach. However, the majority of worksite professionals I have trained and participation data from many companies suggest that many high-risk groups (blue collar, racial, cultural, ethnic populations) are not adequately involved in worksite health promotion activities. This would suggest the need to target your approach to reach these groups in your broader plan and objectives.

Second, the one-size-fits-all philosophy does not work when you consider that all employees are unique individuals with some similar interests but all with different health needs and problems. If you acknowledge that all employees present unique and diverse educational and health situations, you will direct your attention to identifying the activities that would best address their needs.

It makes good marketing sense too. Why would U.S. businesses spend billions each year to market their products to different segments of our population unless they had specific research and sales experience that would support these types of approaches?

The final—and perhaps most important—reason you should consider targeted programs for diverse groups is clear from the disturbingly high morbidity (illness) and mortality (death) rates among these populations.

These same trends will be evident among many of your employee groups and will require some level of special attention and planning. Recall the "epidemiological" model, which public health professionals use to investigate the causes and extent of health problems in any given population and through this analysis are able to target their efforts and resources more effectively to reduce and eliminate the incidence of communicable and chronic diseases.

All these factors should demonstrate the rationale for developing specific **(not necessarily separate)** programs for diverse racial, cultural and ethnic populations. Using the term **separate** is not appropriate because these program services should relate back to the broader diversity program you have developed.

2

The Health Status of Racial and Ethnic Populations: Challenges and Needs

As the face of the American workforce changes to reflect the racial and ethnic diversity of our country, you will want to know the continuing and specific health risks facing different populations.

Here's the picture for the next ten years: By 2005, the labor force—defined as those working or looking for work—is expected to number 151 million, an increase of 24 million from 1992, according to the latest projections made by the Bureau of Labor Statistics. Women are still expected to enter and remain in the labor force at rates faster then those of men (highest among Asian women), yet slower than rates in the past. The baby boomers are aging, but rates for workers ages 45 to 64 are expected to grow most rapidly.

Workers representing racial and ethnic groups are projected to have the strongest growth rates overall. High rates of immigration among Hispanics and Asian and Pacific Islanders especially will add new workers to the labor force.

THE CHANGING WORKPLACE

Projected growth in racial and ethnic groups in the U.S. labor force, in millions

	1992	2005
African Americans	13.6	17.3
Hispanics	10.1	16.5
Asians and others*	4.5	8.2

*The Bureau of Labor Statistics includes Asian and Pacific Islander Americans and Native Americans in this category. From *Monthly Labor Review*, November 1993, p. 32. [1]

Like many health promotion planners, you may have never looked at your wellness program in terms of diversity. And, although you know you should be programming for all employees, maybe you wonder why some never take part. Why haven't you reached them? And what can you do?

As the labor statistics show, the four major ethnic and racial groups are an emerging majority, and this chapter discusses their specific health risks and offers insights into how you can indeed tailor your health promotion program to reach them. For guidance we turn, first, to the nation's health promotion objectives called Healthy People 2000.

Healthy People 2000

The U.S. Public Health Service and other public and private organizations around the country—the Wellness Councils of America among them—helped build the nation's decade-long initiative to meet health promotion and disease prevention objectives by the year 2000. This initiative—known as Healthy People 2000—aims to make the United States a nation of healthy people, regardless of age, race, or socioeconomic status. It builds on earlier efforts begun in the late 1970s to achieve national health goals.

During the 1980s, government objectives for improving clinical preventive services, health protection, and health promotion provided a common strategy and a frame of reference that sparked new initiatives by state and local governments and community organizations. Perhaps most important, these cooperative efforts provided a sense of unity for the various organizations that contribute to the health of the country.

Healthy People 2000 Goals

▌ Increase the span of healthy life for Americans
▌ Reduce health disparities among Americans
▌ Achieve access to preventive services
  for all Americans

To guide the year 2000 efforts, hearings were conducted in seven cities across the country. Nearly 800 health professionals, health-serving organizations, and interested citizens spoke or submitted testimony. The hearings were the first step in a three-year process. In all, 20,000 people were consulted, and a public draft was revised, refined, and published as *Healthy People 2000: National Health Promotion and Disease Prevention Objectives* (see **Sources for More Information** to order this book). Ultimately, 300 objectives were set, and progress is being tracked.

Worksite Targets

Guided by Healthy People 2000, the Wellness Councils of America has set its agenda for the decade by targeting areas where employers can make a difference in the health of the nation. These areas include physical activity, nutrition, tobacco, maternal and child health, clinical preventive services such as screenings, mental health, and occupational safety.

Two objectives define the worksite goals directly:

Increase to at least 85 percent the proportion of workplaces with 50 or more employees that offer health promotion activities for their employees, preferably as part of a comprehensive employee health promotion program (8.6).

In 1985, some 66 percent of worksites with 50 or more employees offered at least one health promotion activity. In an updated survey by the Office of Disease Prevention and Health Promotion in 1992, the number of worksites with health promotion activities increased to 81 percent and nearly met the goal. That's the good news.

Increase to at least 20 percent the proportion of hourly workers who participate regularly in employer-sponsored health promotion activities (8.7).

Although the scope of this companion goal has not yet been measured, according to Healthy People 2000, "Hourly workers have greater health risks and higher rates of illness and injury than salaried workers.

> Contributing factors include socioeconomic differ-
> ences, differences in the nature of the work performed,
> differences in having employer-sponsored health
> insurance, and the exclusion of hourly workers from
> worksite health promotion programs . . . not by intent,
> but by failure to market the program to hourly work-
> ers." Here is where health promotion programs with
> special emphasis on reaching diverse populations can
> make the greatest impact.

The health objectives set forth precise numerical targets, and, for most measures, baseline data were available
for measuring progress toward achieving specific objectives.
However, consistent statistics were difficult to find for
racial and ethnic groups. (Government data often distin-
guish only between the categories of *black* and *nonblack* or
white and *nonwhite.* Therefore, separate data for
Hispanics, Native Americans, and Asians are often simply
unavailable.)

Without data, it's difficult to show the need for health
programs and to direct appropriate health promotion programming. At the same time, many experts testified during
the Healthy People 2000 hearings that health research and
policies fail to differentiate among the special needs of
racial and ethnic communities.

Despite these limitations in data, Healthy People 2000
includes 223 special population targets that address many
of the leading causes of illness and death among racial and
ethnic groups—specifically, African Americans, Asian and
Pacific Islander Americans, Hispanics, and Native
Americans. Although death and disability rates for all these
groups are falling, substantial differences remain.

The gap between white and nonwhite health status in
the United States is so great that Lester Breslow of the

UCLA School of Public Health labeled it "a national disgrace," and he and others called for special attention to reducing [health] gaps in the year 2000 objectives-setting process.[2]

Barriers to Participation

Those testifying at the Healthy People 2000 hearings pointed to the many barriers hindering health promotion efforts among diverse populations, and these included many social, behavioral, and cultural factors; access to health care; and specific health problems of diverse groups. The following discussion summarizes the testimony as reported in *Healthy People 2000: Citizens Chart the Course* (see **Sources for More Information** to order this book). [3]

Social, Behavioral, and Cultural Barriers

Although this book focuses on health promotion in worksites, your employees are significantly affected by quality of life issues in the surrounding community. Issues of employment or fear of unemployment, crime, education, and housing all contribute to the overall health status of individuals and families—the same pool of people from which you draw your workforce. You, as a health promotion professional, must consider how these factors can be addressed within your worksite program.

Poverty. Perhaps the single most important factor affecting the health of the nonwhite population, according to testimony, is poverty. Two to three times as many African Americans, Native Americans, and Hispanics are living in poverty than are whites, according to the U.S. Census. This calculation does not include many working poor or others who subsist just above the officially recognized standards of poverty.

Those living in poor and overcrowded housing are at greater risk of spreading and contracting communicable diseases—for example, tuberculosis is on the rise in poverty-stricken communities. For Asian and Pacific Islander Americans, the tuberculosis rate is nine times higher than it is for whites.

Unemployment. African Americans and Hispanics, as well as other racial and ethnic groups, are disproportionately unemployed. Again, unemployment rates were two or three times higher for Mexican-Americans, Puerto Ricans, Cubans, and African Americans, for example, than for whites. The Indian Health Service reports equally high unemployment rates for Native American men and women. And unemployment rates are even higher if underemployed, discouraged job seekers and youth are included. Among Southeast Asians, unemployment rates can reach as high as 40 percent.

Such high levels of unemployment and underemployment have devastating effects on communities and the health of their members. Unstable economic conditions are associated with crime, general despair, inability to access health care, and stress and can contribute to increased levels of teenage pregnancy, infant mortality, substance abuse, and violence.

Education. Members of some racial and ethnically diverse populations may have fewer years of formal schooling and experience high dropout rates among high school students. Dropouts, in turn, have greater rates of teenage childbearing and substance abuse, and those without education often get trapped in low-paying service industry jobs, many of which do not provide health insurance.

Fewer years of formal education often translates into limited knowledge of health matters and poor understanding of the causes and prevention of disease. For example, in a study of beliefs about cardiovascular disease among African Americans and whites, researchers found that educational level was the most important variable in being able to state the risk factors for heart disease. [4]

In another study, less than 10 percent of Laotians and only about a third of Cambodians knew that smoking causes heart disease, and over 50 percent of Vietnamese incorrectly thought smoking was a cause of tuberculosis. [5] Therefore, efforts to reduce the risks for heart disease among those with less schooling may be difficult, and perhaps the best place to start is with simple education. The fact of the matter is that current medical communication or health promotion efforts in companies tend to offer programs or services that do not account for literacy levels.

Behavior. No one will question the premise that smoking, heavy drinking, use of illegal drugs, and poor eating habits can harm one's health. In many racial and ethnic communities, especially where poverty and low education levels are found, these types of behaviors may be prevalent.

Although there has been much concern over the spread of AIDS through intravenous drug abuse and the onslaught of crack cocaine, experts testifying at the Healthy People 2000 hearings pointed out that the effects of tobacco and alcohol abuse cause disproportionally more death and illness among racial and ethnic groups.

Smoking, for example, leads to a variety of illnesses such as cancer, heart and lung disease, and stroke. Alcohol contributes directly to cirrhosis (liver disease) and cancer. And food preparation practices that are high in fat put African Americans and Mexican-Americans at risk for cancer and heart disease. Asian and Pacific Islander American families seem to be preparing more Western-style high-fat meals, as part of an unhealthy acculturation trend. Traditional diets were lower in fat.

Obesity is especially prevalent among Native Americans, Native Hawaiians, Mexican-Americans, and African American women—putting them at risk for heart disease and diabetes.

Culture. Health promotion professionals may disagree on whether poverty and other socioeconomic differences should or can be targeted in intervention plans or whether race or ethnicity should underlie prevention designs. But for our purposes in this book, health professionals who testified at the Healthy People 2000 hearings did call for "culturally appropriate interventions for minority groups." Such interventions could include recruiting and training health professionals or health promotion planners from the populations they are to serve.

Culture and language are often barriers to health care. Specifically, more than a third of Asian and Pacific Islander Americans do not speak English "very well," and *prevention* may be thought of as a foreign concept. [6] In fact, among all racial and ethnic populations, Asian and Pacific Islander Americans are the least likely to see a physician (42% did not visit a doctor in the last 12 months versus 33% for whites). [7]

No Such Word

"Words English-speaking patients throw around to describe conditions, like hypertension or allergies, often do not have equivalents in languages such as Vietnamese," said Dr. Robert Putsch, University of Washington. The solution: More hospitals must recruit bilingual and bicultural staff and provide interpreters trained in cultural issues. [8]

Access to Health Care

The rules for access to health care are undergoing change. At this writing, we don't know what those rules will be. But let's look at the current situation and draw some conclusions from the Healthy People 2000 testimony.

Because many racial and ethnic populations are more likely to be poor or underemployed or employed without health benefits, they are likely to be uninsured and unable to afford preventive care or any health services. When they do seek medical care, they are more likely to receive it in emergency rooms. Their childhood vaccination rates lag considerably behind those of whites, as do their rates of screening for chronic diseases such as cancer, high blood pressure, and diabetes. Prenatal care may not come until the third trimester of pregnancy.

Furthermore, a sizable proportion of Asian and Pacific Islander Americans, for example, are owners of small, family-owned businesses—grocery stores or restaurants. They, like all small business owners, have an economically difficult time securing health insurance coverage, if it is provided at all, for themselves and their employees.

Some of the racial and ethnic differences concerning access to health services are due to cultural and geographic factors. Many ethnic groups live in areas with shortages of health providers. Inner cities and rural areas, particularly in the South, are medically underserved and have high numbers of African Americans and Hispanics. Therefore, it is even more important for worksites to provide preventive services as part of health promotion programming.

In a Word

The Wellness Councils of America agrees with the editors of the *Los Angeles Times* in defining which terms to use to describe ethnic and racial identification. "It is not important for us to be politically correct," the editors said. "It is important for us to communicate with our readers fairly and accurately."

Therefore, WELCOA has adopted the style of the newspaper and will use *African American* to describe black Americans, keeping in mind that "a black person is not necessarily an African American and that an African American is not necessarily a black person"; *white* not Anglo; *Hispanic* or *Latino; Native American* because the term *American Indian* excludes Alaska Native groups who are not Indians.

Specific Health Problems of Racial and Ethnic Groups

There are nearly 60,000 excess deaths yearly among African Americans, according to the *Report of the Secretary's Task Force on Black and Minority Health*, a landmark study published in 1985 by the Department of Health and Human Services. Although dated in years, the alarming information in the report, according to many respected health promotion professionals, has not changed significantly, and little, if any, substantive progress has been made in serving the health needs of racial and ethnic populations in this country.

The report said, in other words, if African Americans had the same age- and sex-specific death rates as whites, 60,000 fewer African Americans would die each year. These excess deaths have six principal causes:

- heart disease and stroke (cardiovascular disease)
- homicide and accidents
- cancer
- infant mortality
- cirrhosis (liver disease)
- diabetes

Together, these six causes represent 80 percent of the total excess deaths of African Americans. Similar rankings apply for other racial and ethnic groups. Data are not always available to make fair comparisons between death and illness rates of whites and other racial and ethnic groups. If nothing else, this shows how much is still not yet known.

What we do know, however, is that in addition to the six major causes of death and disability cited in the secretary's report over a decade ago, today's discussion must necessarily include HIV/AIDS, tobacco, and alcohol and substance abuse—areas that can be targeted through worksite programs.

Health Profiles

African Americans

African Americans make up 12 percent of the U.S. population and are the largest of the four major racial and eth-

---

Profile information has been excerpted from *Healthy People 2000: National Health Promotion and Disease Prevention Objectives,* where original sources for statistics are cited in full.

nic groups. They live in all regions of the country. Although African Americans are represented in every socioeconomic group, a third live in poverty, a rate three times that of the white population. We know more about the health picture for African Americans than we do for other racial and ethnic groups, except whites, because of the methods used to gather data through surveys.

While life expectancy in this country is at an all-time high, 75.3 years, life expectancy for African American males continued a steady decline and is now only 64.8 years. [9]

The *Report of the Secretary's Task Force on Black and Minority Health* (1985) still reflects the leading causes of death. African American men die from strokes at twice the rate of men in the total population; death rates for African American women from coronary heart disease are higher than for white women. Yet when heart disease rates are compared within income levels, African American rates are lower than those for whites.

African American men have a 25 percent higher risk for all cancers, a 45 percent higher incidence of lung cancer, and a poorer cancer survival rate compared to whites. The key, according to researchers who submitted testimony for Healthy People 2000, was to bring African Americans into treatment at earlier stages and educate them about the connection between certain cancers and behavioral risk factors such as smoking, alcohol use, and diet.

Diabetes is 33 percent more common among African Americans than whites, especially among overweight African American women. They also have twice the rate of blindness as a complication of diabetes than whites.

The rate of AIDS among African Americans is more than triple that of whites, and among women and children, the gap is even wider.

High blood pressure is much more common among African Americans than among the total population, and severe high blood pressure is present four times more often among African American men.

African Americans make fewer annual visits to physicians than whites, and African American mothers are twice as likely as white mothers to receive no health care or care only in the last trimester of pregnancy.

African Americans are six times more likely to lose their sight from glaucoma than whites. Glaucoma is an irreversible disease of the eye associated with a build-up of pressure inside the eyeball.

Smoking rates are 41 percent for African American men age 18 or older and 29 percent for African American women compared with 32 percent for males and 27 percent for females in the total population. As the white community has begun to decrease its smoking behaviors, the tobacco industry has directed its advertising and promotional efforts increasingly toward the African American and Hispanic communities and other groups.

The good news from a 1993 *Gallup Report: A National Survey of Americans Who Smoke,* a study funded by SmithKline Beecham, found that most African Americans (78%) polled say they want to quit and 30 percent are trying to quit. When asked about reasons for wanting to quit, 76 percent cited health problems as a major reason; cost was second (58%); only 23 percent said they wanted to quit because smoking was banned at work. However, restrictive smoking policies and total bans can be effective strategies, especially for smokers who are trying to quit and appreciate the extra motivation.

CHRONIC AND COMMUNICABLE DISEASES FOR WHICH SELECTED RACIAL AND ETHNIC GROUPS MAY DEMONSTRATE A HIGHER LEVEL OF RISK WHEN COMPARED WITH THE GENERAL U.S. POPULATION

	African American	Hispanic	Native American	Asian and Pacific Islander
Heart disease and stroke	●		●	●
Cancer	●		●	●
Infant mortality	●			●
Alcohol and substance abuse	●	●	●	
Diabetes	●	●	●	●
HIV/AIDS	●	●		
Tobacco	●	●		●
Tuberculosis		●		●
Hepatitis B				●

For illustration purposes only.

Adapted from various sources specifically cited in the notes for chapter 2 including the *Report of the Secretary's Task Force on Black and Minority Health,* vol. 1, executive summary; *Asian American and Pacific Islander Journal of Health;* Indian Health Service; Healthy People 2000; *Monthly Labor Review,* November 1993; and National Center for Health Statistics.

Asian and Pacific Islander Americans

Diversity characterizes the more than 11 million people who are Asian and Pacific Islander Americans who speak over 30 different languages and bring with them a similar number of distinct cultures. Their origins are in East Asia (China, Japan, Korea), Southeast Asia (Philippines, Vietnam, Cambodia, Laos, Thailand, Malaysia, Singapore, Indonesia), the Indian subcontinent (India, Pakistan, Bangladesh, Sri Lanka, Burma), and the Pacific Islands (Hawaii, Guam, Samoa, Tonga, Fiji, and other Micronesian islands).

Chinese-, Filipino-, and Japanese-Americans make up 54 percent of this group; Asian Indians and Koreans each account for 11 percent; Vietnamese about 8 percent. Over two-thirds are foreign born (for comparison, 90 percent of Vietnamese were born in Vietnam while just a fourth of Japanese-Americans were born overseas). The largest numbers live in California, Hawaii, and New York in urban areas.

The socioeconomic and health profiles of these distinct people are also diverse. Those born in the United States and established here for generations are similar socioeconomically to the population as a whole. In fact, their median incomes are higher than the overall U.S. population, particularly among Japanese-Americans. Yet some groups, particularly recent immigrants from Southeast Asia, are extremely poor.

Faced with Western medicine and a health care system that is unfamiliar, Americans of Asian heritage experience unique access barriers to primary care. In addition to linguistic and cultural differences, financial problems beset many subgroups, especially recent immigrants.

Thanks to Moon S. Chen, Jr., PhD, MPH, editor of the *Asian American and Pacific Islander Journal of Health,* for providing current statistics for Asian and Pacific Islander Americans. Many of the studies cited here can be found in the journal (see **Sources for More Information** for subscription details).

Heart Healthy Traditional Foods

Among Native Hawaiians, for example, are high rates of heart disease, and stroke—signaled by risk factors such as high blood pressure, obesity, and high cholesterol. By replacing a high-fat Western diet with the Hawaiian diet prevalent in Hawaii before Western contact, the Waianae Diet Program was able to decrease blood pressure, cholesterol, and obesity levels significantly and was a major contributing factor in lowering the number of cases of non-insulin-dependent diabetes. Participants ate taro, poi, fish, sweet potatoes, and other traditional foods instead of high-fat canned meat products and other Western foods that have become popular in Hawaii. [10]

Of great concern for Asian and Pacific Islander Americans is smoking and its implications for lung cancer and heart disease. Acculturation—or the length of time a person is living in the United States and adopts habits of other cultures—can work for health or against it. For example, Southeast Asian men are at very high risk for lung cancer and cardiovascular disease, perhaps because their smoking rates are among the highest at 55 percent (among Laotians the rate is 72%). Although acculturation appears to result in decreased smoking for Asian men, for Asian women, whose smoking rates are relatively low, acculturation appears to result in increased smoking. [11]

High-fat Western diets may be to blame, some studies suggest, for groups that face a high risk for diabetes, including Filipinos, Japanese, and Koreans. By adding more animal fat and sugar to their diets, Chinese-Americans have increased their rates of colon cancer when compared to Chinese in China. Less healthy dietary changes have also occurred among Asian Indians, Japanese-Americans, and Vietnamese-Americans. Stomach cancer is about five times higher among Korean-American men than in white men. Yet knowledge of cancer risk factors and participation in cancer screening is much lower in Asian and Pacific Islander populations, researchers found in comparing groups in California. [12] Obesity and diabetes is also prevalent among Native Hawaiians, where breast cancer is also higher than it is among whites. [13]

Asian Indians have one of the highest rates of heart disease, yet conventional risk factors fail to explain these rates. The higher incidence of insulin resistance and abdominal obesity among Asian Indians may explain why heart disease among these people is three times the rate for the U.S. population. [14]

Tuberculosis is still the leading cause of death in some Asian countries and has become a serious health problem in several Asian communities in large American cities. Among Southeast Asian immigrants, the incidence is 40 times higher than in the total population.

Higher rates of hepatitis B are also found among Asian immigrants. This infection is associated with chronic liver disease, cirrhosis, and liver cancer.

Hispanics

Hispanics—the fastest growing ethnic group—includes populations with origins in Mexico, Puerto Rico, Cuba, Europe, and Central and South America (including Dominicans, Salvadorans, and other Caribbean groups). Two-thirds of Hispanics are Mexican-Americans.

Sixty percent live in the West and Southwest; 50 percent of Cuban-Americans live in Florida. The Hispanic population lives mainly in urban areas, including more than two million in the New York–New Jersey area.

It's a young population with a median age of about 25 years compared to almost 33 for the U.S. population in general. Birth rates are high; yet despite a lack of prenatal care, Hispanic women—and specifically Mexican-American women—have lower infant mortality rates than other groups, including whites. Barriers to care include language differences between Spanish-speaking patients and English-speaking health professionals and costs.

Like many other groups, Hispanics receive less preventive health care. Among the risks to health, smoking continues to be high (43% among Hispanic men).

Obesity is common among Hispanics, especially Mexican-American women. High blood pressure and high cholesterol levels found among Hispanics leads to heart disease. Diabetes is also a risk factor.

Overall cancer rates are lower for Hispanics, yet current data tend to be misleading because Hispanics are less likely to be screened for cancer. Acculturation may also affect these differences.

AIDS has levied a disproportionate toll on Hispanics. The rate of AIDS among Hispanics is more than triple that of whites (more than seven times higher for Puerto Rican–born Hispanics). HIV transmission among Hispanic women is primarily linked to intravenous drug abuse by these women or their sexual partners or to sexual partners who are infected..

Native Americans

Descendants of the original residents of North America now number approximately 1.6 million. More than 500 tribes and bands with their own customs and cultures comprise the American Indians and Alaska Natives. The Cherokee and Navajo are the largest tribes.

About half of the American Indian population live in the Western states of California, Oklahoma, Arizona, and New Mexico; and North Carolina also has a large population, but federally recognized tribes live in more than 33 states. The Indian Health Service provides health care to American Indians and Alaska Natives of federally recognized tribes. About a third of this population live on reservations or in historic trust areas.

Income and educational levels tend to be low, with more than one in four living below the poverty level. This is a young population, but one reason may be that a large number of Native Americans die before age 45. Most of the excess deaths—those that would not have occurred if their death rates were comparable to those of the total population—can be traced to six causes: unintentional injuries, cirrhosis (liver disease), homicide, suicide, pneumonia, and complications of diabetes.

Diabetes has reached epidemic proportions in many tribes. Obesity contributes to the high incidence of diabetes experienced in so many American Indian communities, and it is also linked to high blood pressure and heart disease. Dietary fat intake can also affect obesity.

Cancer rates vary widely among tribes but are lower overall compared to the general population and may be affected by a shorter life expectancy. Yet cancer remains, along with heart disease, a leading cause of death for Native American women, according to the Indian Health Service. [15]

The top two causes of death among Native American men are heart disease and a category the Indian Health

Service calls "accidents." An estimated 75 percent of these are alcohol-related and about half involve motor vehicle crashes. Alcohol is also a factor in suicide and homicide rates that are measurably higher than those of the total population.

Once traditional and socially acceptable, smokeless tobacco appears to be reemerging as a popular form of tobacco use especially among Native American adolescents.

Exercise for Diabetes Control

A community-based exercise and weight control program for the Zuni Indians of southwest New Mexico was designed to help reduce risk for cardiovascular disease and non-insulin-dependent diabetes. Those who participated lost significant weight, and diabetics improved their glycemic control. Weight loss competitions, such as this one, can serve as a model for health behavior change in similar racial and ethnic communities—and in worksites. [16]

Implications for the Worksite

Many of these diseases (heart disease, cancer, diabetes) share common behavioral risk factors. All benefit from early detection and treatment. And worksite programs can be tailored to put special emphasis on these successful types of interventions:

1. **Education and awareness programs** can be conducted using brochures, booklets, and videos (in a second language or with appropriate readability levels, if needed). Worksite health planners will want to call upon speakers representing various racial and ethnic groups to conduct

lunchtime sessions on single topics or to convene small group meetings. Collaborate with community groups and other health-serving organizations in your area. AIDS awareness programs at work can be effective and easy to present.

2. **Primary prevention programs** include smoking awareness (don't start), exercise, and nutrition and diet classes. Invite family members and significant friends to attend along with employees. Group classes or self-help programs are effective techniques.

Worksite programs have the opportunity to provide appropriate prevention and intervention for high-risk pregnant women and their infants—even if the pregnant woman is not herself employed but is the wife or daughter or relative of an employed person who gets information at work.

3. The question of who gets access to care and early **screening** may be far more important in cancer detection and treatment, and worksites can provide such screenings as part of a comprehensive health promotion program. Screenings might involve mini–health fairs held at the worksite, or the employer might reimburse employees who take part in community health screenings at community centers, churches, shopping malls, or hospitals. Again, collaborate with local health departments, community health centers, youth clubs, and other groups who serve your employee populations. Direct intervention with employees at high risk is being used in some companies.

The list of health risks can seem overwhelming, and you and other health promotion planners may wonder where to begin. But, in truth, the course is clear. You begin with your greatest risks overall. If you have a high number of African Americans and Hispanics in your workforce, concentrate on education and awareness programs and screenings in the areas where available health data suggest they are at highest risk such as high blood pressure, cancer, diabetes, and glaucoma. The key is to help all employees know about the ill effects of poor lifestyle choices. In other words, they need to know what is unhealthy. Then help them understand how to make important changes.

It's not that simple, though, and a sound health promotion program will start with a workplan—the subject of the next chapter.

Incentives Boost Participation

Beth Israel Hospital is a Boston teaching hospital with a culturally diverse workforce of over 5,000 employees—10 percent of whom are non-English speaking. In 1991, participants in the hospital's "Be Well! Rebate"—a wellness program designed to provide cardiovascular health screening—would receive $2 per week in additional income if they were making an effort to improve their health. Special efforts were made to reach racial and ethnically diverse groups and non-English-speaking employees.

Of 1,426 participants, 27 percent were considered to be among the targeted group of diverse employees—and 30 percent of these employees were found to be at high risk. Of these high-risk employees, 21 percent lowered one or more risk factors. The conclusion: A financial incentive can attract a significant portion of all employees and, at the same time, motivate them to manage their health risks. [17]

3

The Workplan

How can your organization deliver health promotion services to diverse populations of employees? A solid workplan will help guide your efforts and make evaluation easier. Once you've cultivated senior management support, formed an all-volunteer employee advisory committee, conducted a thorough survey of your workforce using the concepts and strategies presented here, you will want to draft a plan to guide your continuing efforts. This section will take you through that process.

WORKPLAN

Get senior management support
Recruit a voluntary advisory committee
Assess the needs and interests of your
  workforce
Adapt your program to diverse audiences
Test and evaluate a small program

Get Senior Management Support

Certainly, you need strong and significant support from top management—as you would need for any health promotion program. Involvement of senior staff and the CEO is the key to long-term integration of your program for diverse employee groups.

In addition, gain support from top-level managers who are members of racial and ethnic groups represented in your workforce. Also keep key organizers informed and included; these are, of course, union leaders and heads of organizations such as the Black Employees Network at Union Pacific Railroad.

Recruit a Voluntary Advisory Committee

Form an advisory committee that represents the racial, ethnic, and cultural (and gender, age, ability, and other) diversity in your workforce. You need not form a new group if you can tap into an existing all-employee team, or you may restructure a committee that has been formed for other purposes.

Caution: Current committees may not yet reflect the diversity in your workforce. You'll want to follow these guidelines in recruiting or retaining members (and for more information on how an all-employee advisory committee can assist your overall health promotion program, see the Wellness Councils of America's book *Healthy, Wealthy & Wise: Fundamentals for Workplace Health Promotion*).

This group will work with you to establish program priorities, develop specific objectives for the year and beyond, and assist in carrying out activities (such as facilitating discussions, developing appropriate materials, and organizing special events).

Your advisory committee members will, in most cases, be volunteers.

Typically, people volunteer to serve on health promotion committees for the following reasons:

■ They enjoy spending their leisure time involved in sports or fitness activities.

■ They have a personal commitment to health promotion resulting from their own experiences (positive or negative) or through their experiences with families and friends.

■ Their friends or trusted associates are also part of the group.

■ They know and personally "connect" with you or have developed interest in what you have shared with them about the program.

■ The company has offered "incentives" for participation, and the incentive offered is meaningful, of value, or is desirable to them.

It is rare that someone would volunteer to be involved in a committee simply because you asked them to or that it is the "right thing" to do. Usually a personal or individualized reason motivates them to participate.

Using this rationale, in conducting your surveys, focus groups, or other analysis of the worksite population, you should consider asking prospective committee members the following questions:

■ Have you ever volunteered for any special project, group, or activity on the job or in the community? If you have, please describe what the activities were and the single most important reason why you decided to volunteer your time.

- What are reasons why you would not (or cannot) volunteer your time?

- What program, activity, or course would be of interest to you and motivate your volunteering to be a part of it?

- If you knew a good friend, family member, or work associate were volunteering for a program, would that make you more likely to participate?

- What types of gifts, prizes, incentives, or other items have motivated you to join a contest, activity, or program? Please describe them and tell why these items were of particular interest or value to you.

Using these questions and reviewing the responses can help you choose an effective advisory committee. Whom are you looking for? Employees who show **commitment** (they're not volunteering just to get out of work; they have a personal commitment to the company and to living a healthful life themselves), **leadership** (coworkers listen to them and look to them; find the informal leaders and definers), and **availability** (someone who sits on every employee committee may not give yours the time and commitment you need).

A Mirror of the Workforce

Race, ethnicity, gender, age, and occupational status are just some of the factors to consider in recruiting your committee. As a general rule, you want a representative group of people to work with. However, it is important to consider the following issues:

▋ You are advised not to use a "numbers" (or quota) approach in establishing your committee. Make it clear that the group is open to all, and you want everyone to have the chance to participate if they desire. Rotate membership (six months, annually), develop special committees or subgroups to give more employees a chance to participate and to keep ideas fresh. Consider appointing at least two representatives from each racial and ethnic group, if feasible; they will be mutually supportive. And include representatives from other sites (the plant across town, the satellite office in the suburbs, and the office in another city—by conference call).

▋ As you recruit employees to serve on this committee, make it clear that your definition of diversity includes all employees, supervisors, and administrative personnel. You want to create bridges and consensus, not divisions and separation. Often, employers may see the diversity concept as a "minority" or "people of color" program. A true diversity model incorporates all people at different levels with special attention given to individual and group needs and interests. Among Asian and Pacific Islander Americans, for example, deference to the eldest is a custom. Therefore, consider gaining support and approval (and committee involvement) from the eldest Asian and Pacific Islander employee in each ethnic group.

▋ Let your advisory group choose its own title or designation to promote partnership and ownership of the product (your services), its activities, and outcome. Do not establish the name of the committee or advisory group until they have been brought together to discuss the program's goals and objectives.

? *"I am uncomfortable addressing the diversity topic because I am not a person of color and because our company's previous history in areas of affirmative action and equal opportunity employment has had mixed results.?"*

First, diversity is not simply a "person of color" issue. It is everyone's issue and should not be a barrier for you to proceed with the processes outlined in this book.

Second, if you are personally uncomfortable because you feel you lack experience, knowledge, and expertise in this area, you are not alone. All of us are somewhat lacking in dealing with diversity issues, and the key to success is by examining your own personal culture, ethnic identity and being honest, sincere, committed, and responsive to any of the diverse groups you are working with in the company.

Too often people believe they have to "walk the walk and talk the talk" of any group "different" from themselves in order to be accepted. That is a great misperception. Generally people accept (or reject) you because of your personal character, integrity, honesty, and commitment to helping them or working cooperatively on a project or issue. Use these trials to develop trust, respect, insight and cooperation with any culturally diverse group you are responsible for serving in worksite health promotion.

▊ Be clear about what types of roles or responsibilities you would like to see committee members assume in your wellness program. Keep an open mind to all of the committee's suggestions but also have some definite areas where you need their participation and support. Let one of the members be the chairperson. You act in an advisory capacity.

▮ Strongly consider inviting local community organizations or groups as additional members of your advisory committee. Advisers from organizations such as public health departments, human service, and family-centered programs can bring substantial expertise, knowledge, and support for your efforts in working with diverse groups of employees.

▮ Conduct this exercise with your committee: Ask members to think of the term *diversity* and write down on paper their first thoughts. Ask the group to share their impressions and discuss what the term should mean in their workplace health promotion program. Ask the group to draft a mission statement—or modify an existing one—to give meaning to the term *diversity* and how it applies to their work setting and health promotion program (see chapter 1 for guidance in drafting your mission statement). Keep in mind that some members of your group may harbor a one-dimensional or biased view of diversity, and what it means to them can be construed negatively. Explain that you want to redefine the term to include all views, but ultimately the group's goal should be to build consensus around one statement.

▮ Use a problem-solving format to structure the work of the committee. Present and agree on the problem statement. This becomes your constitution. Use it to stick with the work at hand and you won't get sidetracked by committee members who have special interests.

? *"I do not believe I have the budget or staff resources to accomplish many of the crucial activities and tasks. How can I still achieve a quality program that addresses the diversity issue?"*

Creativity, not budget or staff, often times is the solution to achieve many of these program tasks and activities. First, no matter what size your budget, staff, or resources, always think in terms of collaboration and cooperation to design, implement, and evaluate your worksite program.

But, like any business venture or corporate program, you need start-up or operating funds to put programs in place that will, ultimately, achieve long-term savings for the company through your health promotion program. That's your pitch to senior management.

Second, identify program areas or activities which, with proper training and orientation, can be carried out by volunteers.

Third, look into your worksite's surrounding community or area. Are there colleges, universities, health departments, voluntary agencies, service clubs? Many of these groups have the capability of engaging in collaborative activities to supply you with the people power if you supply them with the project or program which fulfills their needs and interests.

Assess the Needs and Interests of Your Workforce

To construct a program model that seeks to meet the needs of all employees, you need to know the makeup of your employee population and their specific health risks. Here's an action plan to find out this information.

Every workplace health promotion manager needs to know whom he or she is serving. It's not always easy to look around and tell by the faces which racial and ethnic populations are represented in your workforce. Your employees may be located in remote sites around the country, in satellite offices across town, or throughout several floors of a skyscraper in New York. Your company may have several plants located in adjoining states.

So how do you find out what your workforce looks like? Of course, the obvious: Ask the personnel department for a profile, but this will just give you numbers. You need to know beliefs and practices, and the best way to gather that information is through surveys and assessments. Here are the kinds of information you will want to ask (and you may adapt and use the sample survey in the appendix):

■ Identify where employees were born and raised. In what region of the United States? From which country did their family or relatives emigrate?

■ In requesting racial, ethnic, or cultural information from your employees, clarify that you are seeking a "self-identified" designation from them. Example: The U.S. Census Bureau used the term *Hispanic;* however, in this category are numerous subgroups representing different regions and distinct cultures: Mexico, Puerto Rico, Cuba, Dominican Republic, Spain, and Latin American countries. This is also true for Asian and Pacific

Islanders, Native Americans, and African American populations. Ask them to be specific.

▌ Employees' lifestyles may be influenced by major political, social, economic, or historical issues. For example, employees who have arrived from other countries with strong totalitarian forms of government may not seek government services. Because of a possible fear of invasion of privacy, they may not take their children to public health clinics for inoculations. Be sensitive to these factors that might have shaped their health attitudes, beliefs, and practices.

▌ Identify previous or current experiences with medical and health care services. If all employees' experiences and doctor visits have been primarily in the treatment of disease and illness, then you have your work cut out for you to persuade them into thinking of prevention or early intervention services. Also, negative experiences with medical and health care professionals can significantly influence employees not to seek care. This may be especially true for employees who are new arrivals to the United States or who are representative of high-risk populations. Frequently, these groups have reported that the handling and treatment of their individual and family health needs have been less than satisfactory. They tend not to go to follow-up visits or seek additional services. Let's say a son or daughter is asked by the physician to translate or interpret health information for a parent who cannot speak English. In some cultures, this may be considered inappropriate, disrespectful, and a violation of the level of status of the parent; thus, the patient may not return for care.

The Power of Tradition

"It is more effective to fit new health information into the old frame of reference than to 'educate' these beliefs away." For examples: "Some Hispanics [Puerto Ricans] believe that health conditions are either 'hot' or 'cold' and that hot conditions should be treated with cold remedies and vice versa. Since pregnancy is considered a hot condition, pregnant women are likely to reject taking vitamins—a hot treatment. The effective approach is to recommend that vitamins be taken with cold fruit juice, a measure that would be perceived as preserving the body's essential hot/cold balance.

"Similarly, in treating some Asian/Pacific Islanders who consider certain herbs as specific for certain diseases, the knowledgeable and sensitive health care provider might recommend that medicine prescribed for high blood pressure be taken in conjunction with an herbal tea." [1]

▪ Ask employees to define in their own words what it means to "be healthy." How have their parents and extended family members addressed health care needs and problems? Do they use nontraditional or home remedies in the family? Again, you are trying to determine how the employees view their health, what has shaped their beliefs, and what things continue to influence their lifestyle or behaviors related to health issues.

Now it's time for you to go to work to fill in the information you need to know about health risks. Here's how:

▪ Examine your worksite demographics and compare these with local, state, and national data.

What specific health risks—as briefly described in chapter 2 of this book—might you find among your employees? Your state may have an agency on minority affairs to provide assistance.

▪ Talk to city and county public health officials including the health officer, epidemiologist, director of public health nursing, maternal/child health director, and the director of health promotion. These people will, to a large extent, be some of the most knowledgeable and experienced professionals in providing you with a detailed description of health problems among the diverse groups in your geographic area. As you are aware, the public health department's primary function is to prevent and control communicable and chronic disease and promote the health of local communities. In other words, if you have a high number of Native Americans in your workforce, and you know that diabetes is a risk factor for them, the public health officials in your city or your local American Diabetes Association may already be doing some community interventions you can plug into. They'll also know if other diseases, such as HIV/AIDS, are reported to be high in your community.

▪ Identify and meet with community-based health centers and clinics. Many of these are providing significant levels of medical and health care services to racially and culturally diverse groups. Their knowledge and experiences in this area would be helpful in constructing your program services.

▪ Contact local, state, and national groups providing health and human service programs for the various racial, cultural, and ethnic populations.

In addition to providing you with any current data or statistics, they may also be conducting health promotion projects addressing issues of relevance to your worksite populations. Look for names and addresses of national organizations in the **Sources for More Information** section of this book.

▮ Ask your company's insurance carrier to provide aggregate reports on the nature and extent of employees' health claims. What are their most frequent health problems? Why are people seeing doctors? Which claims were preventable?

? *"My company wants a culturally diverse worksite health program implemented immediately. How can I address their needs while at the same time properly assess, plan, and develop my own strategies?"*

Give your administration 30-, 60-, and 90-day plans along with broader six- to 12-month workplans that contain measurable short- and long-term goals and objectives. Explain why you are taking this approach to the diversity issue. Provide examples of other companies that have used a similar process with successful results. Develop a list of names of other local companies and key personnel whom you can write to or call to support your position on this process. Use your "marketing" argument. All successful companies market and test their products and services before they mass produce. It saves time, money, resources, and possibly big failures.

Employees' Wants and Needs

How do you know what employees want? You ask them. And the health promotion field has developed many useful surveys that are designed to ask employees what programs they might attend, when they would attend, and what programs they think they need.

Health risk appraisals are a sophisticated way to find out what specific health risks are common in your workforce. These are self-scored or computer-scored assessments of an individual's health risks. The Indian Health Service, for example, uses a specific health risk appraisal for the population it serves. Questions (and output) are specifically tailored to assess the health risks of Native Americans. (Wellness Councils of America's book *Healthy, Wealthy & Wise: Fundamentals of Workplace Health Promotion* contains several needs and interest surveys you may adapt and use in your workplace. This book also contains a lengthy description of how to choose and use health risk appraisals.)

Try to strike a good balance between what employees need and what they want. You'll get the best attendance at those programs. Don't assume that because you have a large number of employees with high blood pressure that they'll attend a program on hypertension. Or that your smokers really want to quit and will pay for a stop-smoking class. Also work with the benefits department to target areas where you have high insurance claim costs. If you see a pattern of high-risk pregnancies and very high-cost deliveries, and your workforce has a large number of young women of child-bearing age, you may want to include questions about prenatal classes on your interest survey.

Adapt Your Health Promotion Program to Diverse Audiences

The key ideas and principles to create a worksite health promotion program that addresses the needs and interests of diverse employee groups will include the following components:

- A **"family-centered" approach** builds on the positive cultural health beliefs of the individual and group, clarifies misinformation, and adds useful, relevant, and practical tips to improve and enhance lifestyles.

- Establish **goals** of team building, sharing achievements, solving problems, and socializing around healthy lifestyle issues. It's easier to lose weight, for example, with the support of your spouse or work group.

- Use food, music, sports, and other significant self-identified cultural events as the means to **promote, recruit, educate, and reinforce health information** and concepts. Soccer, for example, is generally considered a popular sport for certain Hispanic populations (South American and Mexican), particularly among males. Organize activities, programs, and services offering recreation related to soccer, and you may boost your participation in the wellness program.

- **Build on pictorial images,** artwork, literature, language, clothing, or other cultural attributes that reflect the positive of any group's diversity, achievements, and history. These should be incorporated in the worksite health promotion program through multimedia sources (print, audio, visual). Use employee/community residents in leadership roles.

▮ Address **health and human service issues** of interest and relevance to diverse groups of employees. Use national, state, and local health data and research articles related to diverse populations and rely heavily on your own surveys within the employee groups. If glaucoma is a risk factor for your workforce, for example, be sure to include glaucoma screening for all employees at a health fair.

For those managers and staff who are already conducting worksite health promotion activities, here are guidelines for adapting your program to reach more diverse employee groups:

▮ Examine your program's promotional and educational materials (more on developing educational materials can be found in chapter 5). Ask yourself these questions:

Do the pictures, images, or situations portray diversity? (Example: Do brochures show just one racial or ethnic group or several? Be careful not to stereotype.)

Is this material available in more than one language to employees? Does it need to be available in more than one language?

Do the materials acknowledge diversity as an issue in its content? (Example: Are various cultural or ethnic foods discussed in material you distribute about healthy eating?)

▮ Examine your program operations, structure, and delivery system:

Do you make efforts to recruit employees representing diverse backgrounds as participants, team leaders, advisory committee members, or special events planners?

Do you offer services/programs in more than one language?

Do you conduct activities for employees of diverse backgrounds to have opportunities to engage in leadership roles?

Are your programs offered in flexible time schedules? Do you open your programs to family members and significant others?

▍ Review your health promotion program in its relationship with other organizational systems in the company—such as unions:

Is there a defined and specific role for human resources to be involved with your program? For the board or executive staff?

Has your program involved or made efforts to collaborate with employee union groups to enlist their support and participation?

How often have you met with or involved local community organizations serving diverse populations in your program?

▍ Analyze your continuing education of professional staff:

Do you frequently provide staff with materials, research articles, and manuals addressing cultural diversity, health education, and health promotion?

Have you provided any of your staff with an outside speaker who would address managing diversity and its application to your worksite health promotion programs?

Do you attend or send staff to regional or national conferences addressing health and human service issues among diverse populations?

Do you attend events sponsored by community, state, or national organizations that serve diverse populations?

Test and Evaluate a Small Program

Don't overlook the importance of testing and evaluating segments of your health promotion program. In fact, if you start small—and work with smaller groups of employees— you will establish yourself with them and establish your program with company executives. Here are some guidelines:

I Cultivate trusted, respected, and dedicated advocates who will become your spokespersons and role models. This stage of the process requires a great deal of individualized recruitment and interpersonal and intergroup communication to create the dynamics for a successful program.

I Test a small program. You'll spend less money. But carefully identify techniques and strategies that work with your workforce. Eliminate those that don't work. Employees in your company may flock to programs that offer incentives for attending, but try a lunch 'n learn without a door prize, and you might find yourself in an empty room. You'll find out.

▌ Major manufacturers and other businesses test market their products or services to a representative sample of consumers. It makes good business sense to employ this technique, and the most successful companies always place a strong emphasis on this phase of product development and marketing. Use these same techniques with your wellness program.

▌ Work with small groups of employees from various backgrounds. Ask them to help you create the foundation of support you will need to demonstrate health promotion services are available to all groups of employees in the company.

▌ Conduct small group or individualized programs for employees. This creates a less intimidating environment for employees to enter the wellness activities (especially those who are reluctant to attend or never have participated) and allows for them to develop confidence in their abilities to make lifestyle changes.

▌ Testing allows you to build rapport, understanding, and cooperation with diverse employee groups in a more comfortable and productive manner. As the worksite health promotion manager, you need the time, opportunity, and program environment to build and sustain trust and respect from diverse groups of employees.

? *"My company is interested in the bottom line results of any new activity our worksite health promotion program is initiating. How do I satisfy them in this area as it relates to diversity?"*

Begin with the understanding (and acceptance) that in most cases these programs will not quickly change any individual employee's behavior related to their lifestyles. People, regardless of their background, develop a set of personal habits and lifestyles during their childhood and adolescence and sustain these behaviors into adulthood. Your new (or revised) program will not demonstrate an immediate impact in its results if you focus on initially measuring behavior change or create expectations on the part of your management that these will be the results.

Make your case to senior management that your initial evaluation of the program's progress will be a "process" measurement with outcome measures to be established at a later time once employees start regular participation in your worksite activities. Initially, you will assess, evaluate, and report back to senior management on progress in these areas: (1) More and more employees (and more diverse employees) are coming to programs; (2) employees are becoming aware of the importance of making healthy lifestyle choices in their lives.

A long-term evaluation which assesses the outcome of your program activities would involve working with company human resource personnel to analyze individual and group changes in sick days; risk factors such as blood pressure, cholesterol levels, on-the-job accidents, injuries; employee use of preventive as opposed to acute treatment services of your health plan, for examples. I would also encourage you to capture anecdotal information from employees (in writing or on videotape) stating how much of a difference your particular program's activities made in their lives or with their families. Combine the hard numbers and the real-life stories to give a balanced perspective on how well your program is working among employees at your worksite.

Evaluate Your Progress

✓ *What activities, methods, strategies, or materials are most effective among the diverse employee groups?*

✓ *How do diverse groups of employees rate staff and content of classes or the services offered?*

✓ *Has the program been implemented as planned?*

✓ *Are the services and activities reaching a larger percentage of diverse groups than they used to?*

✓ *Can you adapt the program content to meet the needs and interests of diverse employees in your worksite?*

✓ *Can you measure changes in knowledge, attitudes, and health practices?*

These are some of the questions you may want to answer with your evaluation. Finding the answers to these and other questions will be part of your overall evaluation activities. Include, in your evaluation process, how your organization manages diversity and health promotion.

Here are some initial steps to cover as you develop a culturally relevant evaluation component:

▌ Review the public health, medical, social work, and counseling research literature to examine which evaluation designs, data collection methods, and instruments have demonstrated success among diverse population groups similar to those employed in your worksite. Those with access to on-line computer searches can tap into medical databases for this information or contact a library to perform these services.

▌ Check with your local university to determine which departments and faculty have expertise in design and implementation of culturally relevant field studies or evaluation programs.

▌ Identify and contact local, state, or national organizations serving diverse populations and ask for technical assistance and resources related to program evaluation. Many of these national groups can be found in the **Sources for More Information** section of this book.

▌ Contact researchers familiar with conducting evaluations and studies of populations similar to those employed in your worksite. Describe the type of program, activity, goals, and objectives you wish to achieve and ask for their help.

Next, the specific areas you will want to measure will depend on your program needs and evaluation expectations. But, at a minimum, you should examine these broad issues:

▌ The extent to which your health promotion program is serving a more diverse group of employees.

▌ The levels of employee and management awareness regarding the diverse backgrounds and characteristics present in the worksite and how these factors relate to issues of individual risk for disease and disability.

▌ Organizational activities that are being designed and implemented to address the diverse needs, interests, and abilities of employees.

▌ The knowledge, attitudes, and practices of selected groups of employees to determine the levels of their acceptance and incorporation of your program's information related to diversity and health promotion.

As with your overall health promotion program evaluation, these areas should be evaluated using a pretest/posttest methodology that may incorporate written surveys, individual and group interviews, and peer-facilitated discussions. You can use these techniques to get a well-rounded and multidimensional perspective on the effects of your program activities.

This is a basic introduction to program component evaluation. A comprehensive discussion of program evaluation appears in *Healthy, Wealthy & Wise: Fundamentals of Workplace Health Promotion.*

? *"I've tried a so-called diversity approach with some of the employee groups and met with great resistance from them. How can I overcome these types of problems?"*

First, have you properly assessed or determined why there was resistance? Was it you, the program, or the company's sponsorship of it that makes them resistant? Generally, there are some very specific reasons, feelings, attitudes, or perceptions and beliefs held by the resistant group (accurate or not) which have shaped their behavior toward you and the program being offered.

If you can clearly determine these issues, then identify individual employees representative of these groups who may become "allies" or intermediaries on your behalf to work to overcome or reduce resistance. You may also need to work with company administration, human resources, and union groups depending on what problems have been identified. Some issues could involve work grievances or labor relations issues that are certainly out of your realm of direct influence.

Next Steps

The program ideas offered in the next section will help you on your journey.

Given the disproportionately higher incidence of specific chronic and communicable diseases among racial and ethnic populations, it is essential for your worksite program to construct service delivery models that would address their health needs.

A diversity model for workplace health promotion would establish a framework around which you can build services and activities for all employees—with specific targets for those at high risk.

A true diversity model for worksite health promotion services would strike a balance between the needs of all employees and specific identified health risks and problems of racial, cultural, and ethnic groups. The challenge for you is to establish the proper evidence and rationale for addressing specific health needs of subgroups of employees in your worksite and to gain management and employee support and involvement to make it a positive experience for all.

4

Workplan Program Ideas

If you've followed the workplan for health promotion so far, you have gained senior management support, recruited an effective and representative employee advisory group, assessed the needs of the entire workforce with special attention to the diverse groups, adapted your current program or developed new ones, tested a small program, and addressed evaluation design.

Now it's time to look at program ideas. You'll find helpful strategies here for incorporating general health promotion techniques into a plan for reaching diverse audiences.

Once you develop your target areas by assessing employees' wants and needs and by looking at claims data, you will want to build program ideas into your workplan. Consider the following program ideas as a "starter's kit" with the actual long-term plan for your worksite designed in cooperation with your management and employee advisory committee.

Nutrition

▌ Use food service personnel, a community health department nutritionist, or volunteer employees to design culturally diverse menus prepared in "heart healthy" manners (low salt/low fat). Serve some of these items regularly in the company cafeteria. Post calories and fat content and hand out recipes so employees may try them at home.

▮ Demonstrate wok cooking—generally a low-fat way to prepare foods.

▮ Develop and sponsor sessions that instruct employee groups on how to prepare ethnically diverse food choices at home to promote healthier nutritional habits. Fry bread, for example, is a staple in the diet for many Native Americans. It can be prepared in a low-fat manner. You'll be more successful teaching employees how to modify their diets rather than convincing them to change completely.

▮ Give guidelines on how to shop for grocery items and how to compare and select healthier food items. Tailor this program to fit employees' food purchasing, preparation, and economic capabilities. Not everyone uses a microwave, shops in large supermarkets, or can afford to purchase specialty grocery items from a health food store. Take group trips to grocery stores, and teach employees and their families how to read the new food labels.

▮ Publish an all-employee cookbook and include recipe modifications for ethnic foods (or publish a calendar that includes ethnic holidays and recipes for traditional foods). This is an ideal project for your employee advisory committee.

▮ Conduct lunch 'n learn sessions with experts from health-serving organizations such as the American Diabetes Association or American Heart Association who can discuss nutrition and health issues.

▮ Form diabetes self-help groups.

▮ Give advice on how to make canned goods more nutritious by pouring out the liquid and rinsing to eliminate some of the salt. Advise food preparers to boil off fat from soups.

? **"I really want a program or ideas that are quick and simple to implement. Help!"**

This book provides some examples and program ideas that can be implemented in a fairly simple manner. However, achieving a worksite health promotion program that serves the diverse needs of employees takes significant time, effort, and commitment. Anything less will produce average or perhaps inadequate results.

I believe that as a worksite manager, you have an obligation and responsibility to demonstrate to corporate administration that the development and implementation of any program initiated in health promotion takes time to achieve results. Let's view the issue of health promotion in the following context:

If it has taken your employees 10, 15, 20 years to develop specific health behaviors or to establish themselves as high risk for selected diseases, how would it logically follow that one, two, or three years of programming will completely turn their lives around? This is not to say that programs do not have an impact. Rather, we should be more realistic in setting our evaluation of outcome goals with individuals or groups. It does not make sense to establish a belief with your management that dramatic results or change will happen this quickly given these circumstances. The key point to remember is you want to demonstrate that your health promotion program is making positive progress during each evaluation interval (six months, one year, two years) for individuals and groups of employees.

▊ Teach employees how to choose and prepare meals with commodity foods such as cheese. Offer recipes using these food items nutritiously.

▊ Pick a different country or ethnic group each month. Have a food day in which employees bring dishes from that country.

▊ In conjunction with lunch 'n learn workshops on other subjects, ask employees to bring a lunch item from their country of origin. Trade sack lunches, or serve buffet style with samples for everyone. Exchange recipes (try to modify traditional recipes so they are low in fat and salt).

▊ Conduct taste testing in the cafeteria. Food demonstrations are attention getters. Prepare foods in heart healthy ways. Relate food demos to ethnic holidays.

Dieting Needs Company

A new weight control and behavioral modification program specifically designed for African American women is being tested at Baylor College of Medicine in Houston.

"Our earlier study showed African American women benefited from having peers to talk to about weight control and from having a peer to help them learn how to make their lifestyles healthier without giving up important aspects of their culture," said Dr. John Foreyt, director of Baylor's Nutrition Research Clinic. "Our primary goal is not weight loss," Dr. Foreyt said. "We want these women to learn how to take control of their lives and of their weight, to avoid 'yo-yo' dieting and to establish lifelong healthy eating and exercise habits."

Physical Activity

▐ Using diverse groups of employees as your trained volunteer instructors, decentralize your fitness programs and tailor them to individual needs and preferences. Some employees may meet at lunch to walk; another small group might attend aerobic classes after the morning shift at a nearby YMCA; employees in the shipping department might informally shoot some hoops after lunch using the basketball hoop they installed themselves on the dock. Help employees develop an individualized activity plan. You'll get higher levels of participation.

▐ If your company has fitness facilities and offers aerobic or dance programs, incorporate ethnic music and instructors routinely. Try using Native American or other ethnic music in aerobic classes, but do ask a knowledgeable member of the group to select the music. Sacred Native American music, for example, should not inadvertently be used for aerobics.

▐ Conduct culturally diverse fashion, musical, and theatrical performances and slip in messages about fitness, nutrition, and healthy lifestyles. These performances or shows can also serve to reinforce positive messages and images of diverse cultural and ethnic groups as well. Use athletes or celebrities sparingly and preferably as incentives for people to attend these events rather than as role models. Your program's role models should be reflective of the diverse employee groups in terms of culture, ethnic background, socioeconomic level, community environment, and similar life situations.

▐ Sponsor employee teams in recreation leagues. Favorite sports may vary by racial and ethnic group.

▐ National Employee Health and Fitness Day activities (a national event sponsored by the National Governor's

Councils on Physical Fitness and Sports, usually held in May) might be the one event your company (or branch office or site) celebrates as a group—during paid work time—with a walking activity followed by snacks and a recognition ceremony (for your committee members, for employees who have met health goals). Find some way to recognize employees who don't normally receive recognition.

▌ Consider adding tai chi, judo, karate, taekwondo, and others to the company's physical activity programming. Look to your employee base first for qualified instructors.

▌ Organize a demonstration of traditional games or dances (spring is a good time to gather outside, if possible, or in a large space in a warehouse or conference room).

▌ Be aware of any cultural taboos (or discomfort) for some employees if men and women exercise together.

▌ Conduct incentive health trips through countries; walk, run, or bike across a country or continent or around the world; swim or row a river in another country; climb major landmarks (on the stair-climbing equipment or up and down the stairways in the building). Offer appropriate prizes at various stages along the way.

Tobacco Use

▌ Many programs in the public health sector target specific racial, ethnic, and cultural groups to help them stop smoking or not start. In general, your stop-smoking programs for diverse populations should include the following components:

> Self-help materials (audiotapes, pamphlets) with a culturally relevant support group for follow-up composed of other employees who have quit or are in the process of quitting.

Taking the Show on the Road

The men who work on the steel gangs for Union Pacific Railroad are always on the move. They go wherever there are problems with the track and stay until it is fixed. These men (no women) live on the tracks in train cars and are not in one location for long. Now that's a difficult and hard-to-reach population!

Union Pacific has refurbished old railroad cars and turned them into mobile fitness centers. This concept is similar to that of the U.S. Navy which has fitness facilities aboard some of its frigates. The train cars are about 9 feet wide and 54 feet long. The cars contain both strength and aerobic equipment for a complete workout. Some cars are carpeted and have VCR and cable television capability as part of a six-channel individual stereo hook-up system.

Training films and manuals provided from the headquarters fitness center in Omaha are used to educate the crew members on exercise principles and proper use of the equipment.

Unbreakable mirrors provide instant visual feedback, and the exercise graphics printed on the outside of the cars are a symbol of Union Pacific's commitment to wellness. Usage is high, and the gyms-on-wheels have helped boost morale as well.

Information geared to families about health hazards of secondhand smoke and why quitting is important not just for the smoker but also to protect nonsmokers, infants, and children.

▌ Research the history of tobacco and its uses within your various racial, ethnic, or cultural employee groups. In certain Southeast Asian and American Indian populations, tobacco has been used as part of various social events and other cultural ceremonies and traditions. Investigate these issues thoroughly in order to properly address tobacco use issues.

▌ Work to bring about policy changes in the company for designated smoking areas or, preferably, a total ban. Offer smoking cessation classes; consider tuition reimbursement for those who quit and don't resume six months to a year later; open classes to family and friends; don't sell tobacco products on the premises; and offer incentives for those who don't smoke. Make sure smoking cessation classes are available to shift workers (even at the 3 a.m. break).

Stress Management

▌ Create your own program for employees. Rely on information gathered during your assessment phase and in collaboration with local social workers, substance abuse counselors, and school personnel familiar with culturally and ethnically diverse families.

▌ Conduct relaxation exercises for employees using their own cultural/ethnic musical tapes. Provide individual relaxation tapes available in more than one language, if needed, for employee groups.

▌ Modify written evaluations or tests designed to assess life stress events of individual employees. Include culturally relevant measurements. (A good general resource guide published by the federal Office for Substance Abuse Prevention is *Cultural Competence for Evaluators: A Guide for Alcohol and Other Drug Abuse Prevention Practitioners Working with Ethnic/Racial Communities* (see **Sources for More Information**).) Work with university-based ethnic studies departments and local government mental health agencies that have experience designing surveys, evaluations, and instruments that are culturally relevant.

▮ Use traditional stress-reduction methods. For example, many Native American employees who are familiar with the talking circle might like to participate regularly. Encourage this activity and provide a place for it.

▮ Managers and supervisors might be provided with sensitivity training so they can be more understanding and aware of cultural nuances related to stress. Eye contact, for example, may be regarded as rude in some cultures; encouraging competition may be unacceptable for some employees and might lead to job stress. And managers need to know that different cultures have different ways for dealing with stress. The company may be more sensitive to employees who need to use special leave time for ceremonies and other important events not often recognized by the general population.

Concepts of Western Medicine

"For the Southeast Asian, concepts of the world, the human body, reproduction, and illness may counter Western medical practices. The Hmong hold animistic beliefs. They assign meaning and life to natural or organic objects. The significance of spiritual intervention becomes pivotal in successful treatment. The need to draw blood for hepatitis B screening, for instance, intrudes upon these beliefs. Drawing blood is equated with drawing life out of the body. Education which informs the patient about the need for this screening to prevent disease, while respecting the reluctance to give blood, is required for successful health promotion." [1]

Screenings

▋ If the health risk appraisal form you use asks the participant to fill out a section on race or ethnic group, make
sure the criteria for judging health status take into account
the disparity in health risks among various racial and ethnic groups. If you use a health risk appraisal that does not
ask for race or ethnic group, find out why.

▋ Some employees may not be able to read and understand the health risk appraisal. Be sensitive and have
helpers (preferably not coworkers) designated to read and
interpret the questions (in private booths or in another
area). Call upon the free (or nearly free) services of health-
serving agencies to help with screenings in your worksite.
Visiting nurses might be available to help take blood pressure. National blindness prevention groups can provide
screeners for glaucoma and other eye conditions; dentists
for oral cancer checks; podiatrists for conditions of the feet.

▋ Make it possible for any employee at any time to have
his or her blood pressure checked, confidentially, and without fear of being penalized on the job.

HIV/AIDS

▋ Local providers, including the American Red Cross, can
conduct seminars and provide informational materials on
HIV/AIDS. Use posters and brochures; many are available
in various themes and in several languages.

Health Fairs at Union Pacific

Raising awareness is always a challenge among blue-collar workers. When evaluating employee health claims, Union Pacific health promotion managers discovered that the company's blue-collar workers submitted an average of 3.6 health care claims per employee per month. Therefore, the Union Pacific fitness center staff decided to attempt to increase the shop employees' awareness of the benefits of a healthy lifestyle and ultimately to encourage their participation in the company's health promotion program.

They conducted a series of three health fairs in Union Pacific's Omaha and Council Bluffs (Iowa) shops. The fairs were run by the fitness center staff, with help from other health organizations such as the American Heart Association, American Lung Association, American Cancer Society, and paramedic students from a local university.

A month before the fairs were presented, staff contacted the appropriate supervisors to gain their assurance that they would permit their employees to participate, and they posted flyers on bulletin boards in all the shops.

The free health fairs were held in the shops themselves. Eleven stations included screenings, educational material, and test results.

With a 70 percent attendance rate, fitness center staff concluded that this group was indeed concerned about health promotion. They took health services and health information to the target population and made it painless and easy for blue-collar workers to learn about health.

Occupational Safety

▮ Reward employees who buckle up their safety belts with a small token (free muffin in the cafeteria, certificate, box of raisins, chances in a drawing for a larger prize). Catch them as they drive into your company's parking lots (make sure carpoolers are buckled too). And ask those who commute by bus or train. If they say they buckle up when they drive, reward them as well.

▮ Conduct lunch 'n learn sessions on child safety restraints and the importance of using car safety seats for children. Buy car seats and "rent" them to employees who simply can't afford them.

▮ Make it a company policy to buckle up when driving or riding in company-owned vehicles.

Maternal and Infant Health

▮ Explain the family leave act and how it applies to your employees. Some employees may need assurances that they can come back to work after the birth of a child, and you may want to help locate or provide child care referral services in the community.

▮ For many racial and ethnic groups, it's common for extended family members to be living with a nuclear family. Be sensitive to elder care and child care issues.

▮ Hold discussions on cultural values involved in parenting and in the role of the father and what he can do to assist in child care or meal preparation for example.

▮ Educational programs on immunization, childhood illnesses and when to call the doctor are valuable self-care techniques.

▌ Provide a lactation room for breast-feeding mothers and modify leave policies to accommodate their daily needs.

Alcohol and Drug Education

▌ Offer employees the services of an outside employee assistance program. Referrals can remain anonymous, and the employer never knows who has sought counseling and referral for themselves or their family members.

▌ Be open to the idea of holding meetings of Alcoholics Anonymous on company premises or allowing leave time for employees to attend counseling sessions. Make use of traditional talking circles for Native American employees who might attend.

▌ Enforce company policies on alcohol served responsibly at company events or conduct alcohol-free events.

Related Health Issues

▌ As the workforce ages, many employees will be concerned about retirement issues and financial planning. For other employees, just getting to the next paycheck is of primary concern. Set up financial planning seminars—in groups followed by individual counseling.

▌ Don't assume employees understand their health benefits—especially if your company changes carriers or modifies your health plan. Conduct educational forums to explain PPOs, HMOs, deductibles, preventive care, precertification, copayments, and other insurance terms that cause confusion.

Responsible Drinking? How?

During the last two decades, phrases such as "drink in moderation," "drink responsibly," and "know when to say when" have been widely promoted in American business and industry.

The fact of the matter is that up to 47 percent of industrial injuries and 40 percent of industrial fatalities can be linked to alcohol abuse and alcoholism. Problem drinkers are absent from work about four to eight times more than other employees. And untreated alcoholism is associated with higher health care costs and higher premiums paid by companies.

Employers are looking at stronger risk management policies that clearly prohibit drinking by employees who are on duty, who may be called to duty, or who are operating any equipment owned or leased by the company. Although these strategies help to reduce the likelihood of accidents and injuries at the worksite, many alcohol-related problems occur as a result of employees' consuming while off duty and away from the worksite.

Many employers are encouraging their employees to "drink responsibly" when they are off duty. Can it be done, and what is "responsible drinking"? It can mean almost anything from total abstinence to not falling over the cat when tiptoeing in from a late night drinking bout. Also, responsible drinking implies that those who do not drink responsibly drink irresponsibly. This is a judgmental way of characterizing the alcoholic as an irresponsible person. The blame is placed on someone who has an already misunderstood illness. Employees with alcoholism, try as they will, cannot drink responsibly.

At the same time, responsible drinking implies that a person consumes at least some alcohol. In certain situations, any alcohol may be dangerous (such as driving, operating machinery, and pregnancy). And some groups of people should never drink under any circumstances (those with a family history of alcoholism or those with certain chronic health conditions, for example).

So: Is there such a thing as responsible drinking? Health experts suggest that it is possible for those who do choose to drink to substantially reduce their risk for experiencing alcohol-related problems. The Alcoholism and Drug Abuse Council of Nebraska has developed a public information campaign entitled *Reducing the Risk for Alcohol-Related Problems: By the Numbers.*

It's an easy-to-remember alcohol use formula, based on research, to provide employers and employees with more specific guidance in alcohol use: O-1-2-4

ZERO represents no alcohol use. Some people choose not to drink at all. For others, zero alcohol use is the best choice in certain situations such as a family history of alcoholism, medication interaction, pregnancy, or if drinking violates existing laws, policies, or personal values.

For individuals who choose to drink: ONE stands for no more than one standard drink per hour. TWO stands for no more than two drinks per day for men, one for women. FOUR stands for drinking on no more than four days per week.

When worksite health promotion managers are asked, "How much is too much?" or "What is responsible drinking?" this formula may provide a guideline. Certainly this information may help employers make policy decisions about the appropriate use of social controls regarding alcohol in the workplace and in developing company alcohol-use policies.

By the Numbers public education campaign is a copyrighted program used here with permission from The Alcoholism and Drug Abuse Council of Nebraska.[2]

▌ Publish regular columns in the company newsletter about benefits—particularly health benefits and how to be a better consumer of health insurance. Teach employees how to talk to their doctors and when to seek medical care.

▌ Have doctors or other health professionals role play as patients and employee/patients as doctors to illustrate the difficulties of patient-provider communications. Have fun with this, but the point is vital.

▌ Be sensitive to the health concerns of an aging population. They will be interested in information on fractured hips, osteoporosis, menopause, and prostate problems.

▌ Discuss organ donation and living wills and be sensitive to cultural taboos about death and dying.

▌ Organize a company-wide cadre of regular blood donors. Again, be sensitive to culturally based concerns about blood donation.

▌ Consider the cultural implications of gifts or incentives for any program. To give a clock, for example, to a Chinese person is equivalent to wishing death for him or her. Similarly, Chinese do not give knives to each other.

Viewing Life Through a Different Lens

"Procuring organs for transplantation in a quantity that is sufficient to meet the demand is a challenge made even greater by the variety of cultural norms that coexist in the United States. . . .

"The tools to meet this challenge have very little to do with medicine. Rather, they involve the ability to view organ donation through a cultural lens, using understanding and sensitivity to each ethnic group's cultural framework and the ways in which it may influence their decision about whether to donate.

"After the death of a child [in a Hispanic family], for instance, a donor procurement coordinator may go to the father to request organ donation, assuming that, as head of the household, he would make the decision. Yet it is the mother, and especially the grandmother, in most Hispanic families who makes decisions regarding health and sickness. Furthermore, English-based law recognizes the spouse as next of kin. Yet the Hispanic culture, which is descended from collective, tribal groups, determines next of kin by blood. The opinion of the deceased's parents, therefore, would weigh more heavily than the spouse's in the donation decision."

Requests for organ donation can be made in a way that respects cultural differences, and much of this involves understanding the family structure. [3]

Lessons for the worksite: Invite an organ procurement coordinator to your workplace for a lunch 'n learn workshop. Encourage employees to discuss the subject with their family members and learn their wishes.

5

Designing Educational and Resource Materials

Busy health promotion professionals appreciate having access to program materials. This might include off-the-shelf programs that come with employee education videos, posters, handouts, and a trainer's guide. There are many worthwhile programs available, and more and more health-serving organizations and for-profit companies are producing such materials.

In the **Sources for More Information** section that follows, you will find a wealth of information about prepackaged programs, pamphlets, videos, fact sheets, and books that will serve your program well. Many of these resources are available free or at low cost through government sources.

Other health planners will want to develop their own materials—working, of course, with their employee advisory committees. Whether you choose to review prepackaged programs or develop your own, you will want to use these guidelines.

To develop print, audio, or visual materials for diverse employee groups, consider the following process:

▌ Fully assess (written, verbal) your audience's preferences for receiving information that is educational or for entertainment purposes. Do they read newspapers or magazines? Which ones? Do they listen to radio programs for news, sports, music? What are the most popular television programs they watch?

▌ Review cultural/ethnic media sources in the community. In most local areas, there are newspapers, radio, and television stations serving specific racial, ethnic, and cultural groups—often in many different languages. Meet with media representatives of these stations to learn more about how they successfully market their programs, special events, news, entertainment, sports, and health information programs. Enlist their aid in developing your materials. And don't be afraid to ask known media personalities to be spokespersons or promoters of your worksite program.

▌ Contact local school districts responsible for teaching children of your employees. Frequently, they have had to adapt their materials, programs, and services to meet the needs of diverse populations. Adult education programs are good resources particularly those that teach English as a second language. These instructors have had significant experience working with culturally diverse populations. Bear in mind that English fluency is not a measure of education. Persons professionally trained in other countries are well educated—they simply may not speak English well.

? *"My worksite has a significant number of employees for whom English is their second language. I only speak English and find it difficult to communicate and work with these employee groups. Our budget restricts my ability to hire staff capable of speaking this language. How do I address this problem?"*

Identify employees among these groups who are bilingual and bicultural with abilities to speak, write, and translate. Invite them to become a major contributor to your program by offering to train and direct them with health promotion activities for non-English speaking employee groups. Offer them incentives for their leadership (award certificates, free dinner coupons for their family at a local restaurant, tickets to sporting events).

Examine your local community surrounding the worksite to identify which government and private organizations have the human resources available to help you in working with these employee groups. Public health departments, county or city hospitals, and community-based organizations with a recreation component (Boys and Girls Clubs, YM/YWCA) frequently have staff with second language abilities and are trained in health and fitness activities.

▌ At a minimum, the media, images, and methods used to communicate with and educate employees should reflect the differences present in the workforce. For example, you may choose to present educational brochures on high blood pressure in several languages. You will want to make sure employees who might be visually limited or hearing impaired can attend workshops (provide materials in Braille or on audiotape; use the services of a person trained in sign language). Adjust a walking program so employees who use wheelchairs can substitute chair exercise for walking miles, for example.

▌ Those who represent the program or provide services should reflect the differences present in your workforce. Images in brochures, on posters and bulletin boards, and in flyers and table tents should "look like" your workforce yet not stereotype.

If you specifically design print materials for employees who cannot read or who have difficulty reading English, you will want to know about the following strategies:

▌ Use illustrations or pictures with one single, simple message. Illustrations or pictures should represent individuals or groups to whom you are communicating the health messages.

▌ Limit the number of pages. And keep all concepts and information in an order that seems logical and sequential to your audience. Test your materials by designing a sample copy for distribution to employee groups. Provide space on each page for comments and feedback. Ask them if they understand the health concepts and messages. Is the material culturally relevant, and does the reader identify with the illustrations? See the box on the next page for sample questions to ask your test groups.

Lost in the Translation?

Try these sample questions with a focus group of employees from various ethnic backgrounds. See if your own written materials (or materials you might use or buy) are effectively conveying health messages:

1. What information is this page trying to convey?
2. What does the text mean in your own words?
3. If there is a picture, what does it show? Is it telling you to do anything? If yes, what?
4. Do the words match the picture on the page? (Why or why not?)
5. What do you like or dislike about this page?
6. Are there any words in the text you do not understand? Which ones? (If so, explain the meaning and ask respondents to suggest other words that can be used to convey that meaning.)
7. Are there any words that you think others might have trouble reading or understanding? (Again, ask for alternatives.)
8. Are there sentences or ideas that are not clear? (If so, have respondents show you what they are.) After explaining the intended message, ask the group to discuss better ways to convey the idea.
9. Is there anything you like or dislike about this booklet—use of colors, kinds of people represented, choice of foods used, for example?
10. We want the materials to be as good as possible and easily understood by others. How can we improve the pictures?
11. What other suggestions do you have for improving this material—pictures, words, or both?

From *Developing Health and Family Planning Print Materials for Low-Literate Audiences: A Guide* published by PATH. Used with permission. [1]

▌ Text should be simple. Use short sentences and active rather than passive language. Use positive images for illustrations, and select artists who represent the cultural or ethnic employee groups to produce the visuals. (See the sample checklist on the following pages. It's simple, easy to read, and conveys important information. And it's free from copyright, so you may reproduce and use it.)

▌ Review and emphasize important concepts as part of all print materials developed and distributed.

▌ Use employees who are familiar with other languages to translate materials. Written materials should not be simply translated without understanding what terms or phrases are appropriate in different languages. For example, the term *wellness* does not exist in the Spanish language, so another term would need to be identified to convey the same concept. Local universities or college foreign language departments can also help identify appropriate words or phrases to use for educational materials and how to frame the messages—not just translate them. They can also share what kinds of words, phrases, or illustrations might be offensive to the specific cultural or ethnic groups you intend to reach with your materials.

▌ Use your employee advisory committee or employee translators to review newsletters from outside sources that are available in Spanish, if you have a need. Several of the popular health newsletters are available in Spanish, and many large companies buy copies for distribution to their Spanish-speaking employees. Decide how you will ask

Bilingual and Bicultural

"Once people do have insurance, they can't always make use of the services that are available. The services may be across town, or they may be intimidating, or they may not be bicultural or bilingual.

"Keep in mind that making a health service bicultural means more than translating a brochure. It means the staff is bilingual and bicultural; the posters around the room are something the people understand. It means the clinic is located in the community, and the hours are such that people can come in on weekends and at night."

Jane Delgado, PhD, President and CEO, National Coalition of Hispanic Health & Human Services Organizations (COSSMHO),

employees, with appropriate sensitivity, if they would like to receive the newsletter in Spanish, and then decide if you want to mail it to them at home. Home mailings almost guarantee that family members will read the newsletters too.

▌ Check with your local health department and community-based organizations serving culturally diverse populations. Many of these institutions have been the "traditional" providers to diverse families for health, education, and human services. Frequently, they have had to develop appropriate educational materials on a variety of topics—many of which can be related to your health promotion program needs.

A CHECKLIST TO HELP YOU REDUCE YOUR RISK FOR DISEASE
Look for the diseases you are at risk for:

If You Are a Hispanic American...You Are at Higher Risk for:

High blood pressure
Diabetes

If You Are a Black American...You Are at Higher Risk for:

Heart disease
Stroke
High blood pressure
Diabetes
Cancer
Cirrhosis of the Liver

If you are an American Indian or Alaskan Native...You Are at Higher Risk for:

Heart disease
Malignant neoplasm
  (cancerous tumor)
Accidents
Chronic Liver Disease
Cirrhosis
Diabetes
Pneumonia/influenza

If You Are a Pacific/Asian American...You Are at Higher Risk for:

Heart disease
High blood pressure
Diabetes
Cancer

 Check the diseases you are at risk for and try some of the healthy behaviors that may reduce your risk of disease:

❑ Heart disease

❑ Get your blood pressure checked regularly. If you have high blood pressure, keep it under control by limiting salt in your diet and following your doctor's advice.
❑ Quit smoking.
❑ Lose weight by cutting down on fat and calories in your diet.

❑ Get your blood cholesterol level checked. If you have high blood cholesterol, limit fat, especially saturated fat in your diet and follow your doctor's advice.

❑ Get your blood sugar checked for diabetes. If you have diabetes, keep it under control.
❑ Exercise

❏ Stroke

- ❏ Get your blood pressure checked regularly. If you have high blood pressure, keep it under control by limiting salt in your diet and following your doctor's advice.
- ❏ Quit smoking.
- ❏ Get your blood cholesterol level checked. If you have high blood cholesterol, limit fat, especially saturated fat in your diet and follow your doctor's advice.
- ❏ Get your blood sugar checked for diabetes. If you have diabetes, keep it under control.
- ❏ Lose weight by cutting down on fat and calories in your diet.
- ❏ Exercise

❏ High Blood Pressure

- ❏ Exercise.
- ❏ Try to lose weight by cutting down on fat and calories in your diet.
- ❏ Cut down on salt in your diet.

❏ Diabetes

- ❏ Limit sugar in your diet.
- ❏ Control your weight; lose weight if you need to by limiting fat and calories in your diet.
- ❏ Exercise.
- ❏ Drink less alcohol.

❏ Cancer

- ❏ Quit smoking.
- ❏ Cut down on fat, especially saturated fat in your diet.
- ❏ Drink less alcohol.

❏ Malignant neoplasm (cancerous tumor)

- ❏ Quit smoking.
- ❏ Drink less alcohol.

❏ Accidents

- ❏ Drink less alcohol.
- ❏ Check your home for safety risks.

❏ Chronic Liver Disease

- ❏ Drink less alcohol.

❏ Cirrhosis of the liver

- ❏ Drink less alcohol.

❏ Pneumonia/influenza

- ❏ Eat a balanced diet.
- ❏ Drink less alcohol.
- ❏ Quit smoking.
- ❏ If you have diabetes, keep it under control with diet and follow your doctor's advice.

USED WITH PERMISSION FROM
THE NATIONAL RESOURCE CENTER ON
HEALTH PROMOTION AND AGING--AARP

? *How should I start?"*

You should start at two levels. The first is with employee groups you are already serving, and the second is with company executives and management staff. You must simultaneously begin the assessment and examination process with both groups in order to demonstrate program progress with employees and gain support and assistance from management.

Set a meeting with your supervisor, director, or manager to discuss the concepts of diversity as they relate to workplace health promotion and in the context of the organization as a whole. Pledge to begin in very small but measurable steps to determine administration and employees' thoughts, attitudes, and beliefs about diversity. You may want to consider using an outside consultant to facilitate discussions or conduct organizational surveys about this issue. If budgetary resources won't permit this, then consider contacting groups such as The American Institute for Managing Diversity to determine when they are offering training sessions on this subject in your city or state.

If you have an existing advisory committee for your worksite program, initiate discussions about the issue of diversity with them. Consider adding local community organizations and their representatives to contribute their perspective on this topic.

Set timetables for reaching specific milestones in one-, three-, six-, or 12-month periods. For example: Within 30 days, I will have completed the following tasks:

(1) Contacted at least three local health organizations serving diverse populations and conduct meetings on the subject of diversity and health promotion;

(2) Conducted one advisory committee meeting to explore diversity as it relates to the worksite program and the organization as a whole;

(3) Met with my supervisor and company management to determine their thoughts and ideas regarding diversity and health promotion.

Your timetables should reflect a realistic and achievable set of goals and objectives based on your own capabilities, other staff, or that of your organization.

I highly recommended that you take considerable time to examine the diversity issue with your company and determine what you can accomplish given your resources. It's a major undertaking to transform a worksite program that has been reaching a small or limited segment of workers to one that seeks to meet the needs and interests of all employees. Always consider that the idea of managing diversity might be the right idea but not the appropriate time for your company.

6

Sources for More Information

What next? Certainly you will want to find out what resources are available in your own community and in your industry. Here are some places to start and some strategies for finding the best information for your workforce.

▌ Write to some of the organizations listed here. Describe your worksite, job responsibilities, and your wellness program. Ask for assistance. Frequently, these organizations can tailor their resource materials or technical assistance based upon a complete and accurate description of your needs.

▌ Prior to purchasing any educational guidebooks, training manuals, or video programs, request a copy for review. You want to be sure the information you purchase will be useful for your specific worksite program and training needs. (Remember to "test" or "preview" these materials with employees and your advisory committee members.)

▌ Write to authors or publishers asking more specific questions or for updated information they may be working on in the areas of diversity and health promotion. They may be able to put you on a priority mailing list for new articles, papers, or publications to be issued in this area. Subscribe to relevant professional journals.

■ Get your name on mailing lists for national, state, and local groups and associations that are addressing diversity issues.

RESOURCES

Although certainly not all-inclusive, the following listing of organizations and publications, videos and consumer guides, is intended to give readers a way to take the next step. Write or call for more information and educate yourself about the health issues and health risks of employees in your workforce.

Alcoholism and Drug Abuse Council of Nebraska, (402) 474-0930.

> Call for more information about the educational program called *Reducing the Risk for Alcohol-Related Problems: By the Numbers.* Peer-led or video-based modules define responsible drinking and provide an easy-to-remember alcohol formula with specific guidance in alcohol use for employers and employees.

American Association of Retired Persons (AARP), 601 E St., NW, Washington, DC 20049.

> Extensive catalog includes guide called *Celebrating Diversity: A Learning Tool for Working with People of Different Cultures* and booklets on health risks and preventive care among older African Americans, Native Americans, Hispanics, and Asian and Pacific Islander Americans. Write for a catalog.

American Cancer Society, contact your state division by calling (800) ACS-2345.

> Wide variety of materials on cancer, cancer prevention, treatment, and smoking. Ask for a publications list, if available. Single copies of all publications are free; minimal cost for multiple copies.

American Diabetes Association, National Center, 1660 Duke St., Alexandria, VA 22314; (800) ADA-DISC.

> Contact your state affiliate or the National Center for a copy of the Healthy Living catalog of publications. Some consumer information brochures on managing diabetes and nutrition are available in Spanish, and programs for Hispanic, African American, and Native American groups are offered in some locations.

American Dietetic Association, see **National Center for Nutrition and Dietetics.**

American Heart Association, contact your state or local affiliate.

> Consumer pamphlets are available on high blood pressure in African Americans, and several pamphlets are printed in Spanish. Also, local affiliates distribute the *Eating for Healthy Tomorrows* kit—a complete two-hour nutrition education program that encourages lifestyle change. Curriculum can be adapted for use in worksites. Modestly priced, includes slides, handouts, leader's guide, and heart-healthy recipes adapted from traditional African American, Hispanic, Asian, and Native American dishes. Ask for a publications catalog.

American Indian Health Care Association, 245 East Sixth St., Ste 499, St. Paul, MN 55101; (612) 293-0233.

A national membership organization serving Native people in tribal, Indian Health Service, and urban settings. Major emphasis on wellness and prevention. Products include modestly priced self-help guides, brochures, and posters on smoking and AIDS. The *Promoting Healthy Traditions Workbook: A Guide to the Healthy People 2000 Campaign* emphasizes an Indian-specific planning model (Circle of Community Wellness) and is a comprehensive source for further information and strategies. AIHCA publishes a newsletter for health professionals—*Native NewsBriefs.* Call or write for an order form.

The American Institute for Managing Diversity, Inc., 351-55 Westview Drive, SW, Box 38, Atlanta, GA 30314; (404) 756-1170.

The American Institute for Managing Diversity, Inc. (AIMD) at Morehouse College has positioned itself as a national education and research institute in the field of managing diversity. AIMD is helping the general public clarify their vision, strategies, and goals as they relate to managing diversity. The primary focus is research and education. Research includes basic, applied, and action components. The action research focuses on the application of managing diversity concepts within different organizations. AIMD has devoted a number of years researching the elements of organizational culture. The work is made available to the public through a number of education mediums: public seminars, books, videotapes, audiotapes, speeches, conferences/symposiums, monographs, research report findings, in-house educational seminars, and presentations. Call or write for more information.

American Journal of Health Promotion, 1812 S. Rochester Road, Ste 200, Rochester Hills, MI 48307-3532; (810) 650-9600.

> The largest peer-reviewed journal devoted exclusively to health promotion. Formed in 1986, with an editorial board of over 140 of the most notable health professionals in the field, the journal is published six times a year ($59.95/year).

> The Robert F. Allen Symbol of H.O.P.E. Award is given each year at the annual conference to recognize an individual who has made a significant contribution to serving the needs of underserved populations or to promoting cultural diversity within health promotion.

American Lung Association, contact your local branch by calling (800) LUNG-USA.

> Many educational materials available for racial and ethnic audiences on lung disease, tuberculosis, asthma, and smoking, among others. Single copies free; minimal charge for multiple copies for use in worksites. Some brochures available in Spanish.

American Red Cross

> Contact your local chapter for HIV/AIDS prevention education courses specifically taught for Hispanic and African American populations, and those who work with these groups. Red Cross–trained instructors are available to teach HIV/AIDS classes in worksites. Health promotion professionals may also become trained to present the HIV/AIDS program in worksites. Booklets, videos and posters on HIV/AIDS are available as are culturally adapted

emergency services brochures (many are published in Spanish).

Asian American and Pacific Islander Journal of Health, 5525 Corey Swirl Drive, Dublin, OH 43017-3057; (614) 766-5219.

The premier journal dedicated to the scholarly exam-ination of health issues affecting Asians and Pacific Islanders with a multiethnic and multidisciplinary focus. Edited by Moon S. Chen, Jr., PhD, MPH, who previously served as a regional consultant to Johnson & Johnson Health Management, Inc., and has consulted for organizations such as the Centers for Disease Control, the National Institutes of Health, and state departments of health. The peer-reviewed journal, with distinguished and representa-tive boards of advisers and editors, is published quarterly. Subscriptions are $60/year.

Asian American Health Forum, 116 New Montgomery, Ste 531, San Francisco, CA 94105; (415) 541-0866.

National coalition of health professionals, organiza-tions, and others who seek to identify significant health issues facing Asian and Pacific Islander com-munities.

Association of Asian/Pacific Community Health Organizations, 1212 Broadway, Ste 730, Oakland, CA 94612; (510) 272-9536.

A national, nonprofit membership organization rep-resenting the needs and concerns of community health centers serving Asian and Pacific Islander communities throughout the United States. Resources available: *Behind the Mask: AIDS... It Affects All of Us*—a video on AIDS in several languages including Cantonese, Cambodian, Laotian, Mandarin, and Tagalog; brochures, in seven different languages, on childhood illnesses and hepatitis B.

Baylor College of Medicine, One Baylor Plaza, Houston, TX 77030.

Brochure: *Diabetes: We Care for You.* One copy free in English or Spanish. Send stamped, addressed envelope.

California Department of Health Services and the Multi-Ethnic Steering Committee for Health Promotion, (916) 322-6851.

Task Force Reports on the Year 2000 Health Promotion Objectives and Recommendations for California. May 1992. Four separate task force reports outline the Healthy People 2000 priority areas, objectives for each racial and ethnic group, and recommendations for achieving them. Emphasis on community interventions and policy, but worksites may benefit from ideas. Copies free while supplies last.

Health Promotion at Work in California: An Employer's Guide to Assessing Quality in Worksite Health Promotion Programs. One copy free while supplies last.

Center for Science in the Public Interest, 1875 Connecticut Ave., NW, Ste 300, Washington, DC 20009-5728; (202) 332-9110.

A nonprofit consumer advocacy organization that has led efforts to improve alcohol policies regarding labels and warnings on alcohol beverage containers and advertising including billboards targeted to African Americans and Hispanics in particular. Publishes books, posters, and a video. Call for a publication listing.

COSSMHO—National Coalition of Hispanic Health & Human Services Organizations, 1501 Sixteenth St., NW, Washington, DC 20036-1401; (202) 387-5000.

A private, nonprofit organization that seeks to improve the health and psychosocial well-being of Hispanics. COSSMHO provides national leadership and works primarily with community-based organizations in targeting specific health problems, conducts national demonstration programs, coordinates research, and serves as a source of information. Call or write for a listing of publications, videos, and other materials on nutrition, HIV/AIDS prevention, and parenting. Of special note: *Delivering Preventive Health Care to Hispanics: A Manual for Providers*, also *Proyecto Informar,* a training package to improve delivery of health care to Hispanics.

Dairy Council, Inc., 1225 Industrial Highway, Southampton, PA 18966; (215) 322-0450.

Video training program called *Barbershop Talk: Benny's Advice on Healthy Eating* is targeted to African American men and discusses high blood pressure, fatty diets, lactose intolerance, food groups, soul food, and weight control in a familiar setting. Ideal for brown-bag lunch workshop. Video (12 minutes), leader's guide, and 25 participant cards are $15 plus $5 shipping, prepaid. Call or write for information and an order form.

Gallup Report: A National Survey of Americans Who Smoke.

For a free survey briefing book, call Porter-Novelli (212) 315-8144 or fax your name and address to (212) 315-8101. Survey funded by SmithKline Beecham, 1993.

Health Literacy Project of the Health Promotion Council of Southeastern Pennsylvania, 311 South Juniper St., Room 308, Philadelphia, PA 19107; (215) 546-1276.

Education materials (videos, pamphlets, audiotapes) focus on risk factors and behavior contributing to heart health and other health behaviors such as smoking, obesity, and stress and explain diseases such as high blood pressure and diabetes. Materials target African Americans and Hispanics with limited literacy skills and are written at a fourth to sixth grade reading level. Pamphlets—tested for cultural sensitivity, clarity, and appeal—are available as copier-ready masters with space for your logo. Teaching guides are included. Write or call for an order form.

Healthy People 2000: Citizens Chart the Course. National Academy Press, 2101 Constitution Ave., NW, Washington, DC 20418; (800) 624-6242.

Summary of testimony from over 800 national leaders in health, business, and social services who helped shape the nation's health objectives. Much of the testimony comes from the 300 national organizations—Wellness Councils of America among them—and state health departments that make up the consortium on the year 2000 health objectives. Michael A. Stoto, Ruth Behrens, and Connie Rosemont (editors), 1990, $24.

Healthy People 2000: National Health Promotion and Disease Prevention Objectives, U.S. Dept. of Health and Human Services, Public Health Service.

Healthy People 2000 is the product of a national effort, involving 22 expert working groups, a consortium that has grown to include 300 national organizations—WELCOA among them—and all the state health departments and the Institute of Medicine of the National Academy of Sciences, which helped the Public Health Service to manage the consortium, convene regional and national hearings, and receive testimony from more than 800 individuals and organizations. After extensive public review and comment, involving more than 20,000 people, these specific objectives, including targets for special populations, were revised, refined, and compiled in these documents. See also **Office of Disease Prevention and Health Promotion.**

The full report (1990) (stock no. 017-001-00474-0) and a summary report (stock no. 017-001-00473-1) are available from the Superintendent of Documents, Government Printing Office, Washington, DC 20402-9325, call order-and-information desk to verify prices (202) 783-3238.

March of Dimes, 1275 Mamaroneck Ave., White Plains, NY 10605; (914) 428-7100.

For more information on *Babies & You: A Prenatal Health Program*—a health education program designed to reach adults in the workplace with vital information on preventing low birthweight.

McDonald's Nutrition Information Center, McDonald's Corporation, McDonald's Plaza, Oak Brook, IL 60521; (708) 575-FOOD.

> *Convenient Eating Can Be Healthy Eating,* a brochure targeted to African Americans, offers tips for eating on the go, especially for consumers with questions about diabetes, high blood pressure, and high cholesterol.

Metropolitan Life, Health & Safety Education Division, One Madison Ave., New York, NY 10010-3690; (212) 578-5668.

> The MetLife Healthy Living™ Program offers a variety of wellness materials and services from its Stay Well series of pamphlets to its Healthy Living™ question-naire survey—all of which are intended to enhance a wellness program. Professional staff can assist with needs assessment and program development. Write or call for a descriptive kit with catalog and price list.

Minority Health Resources Directory, ANROW Publishing, 1700 Research Blvd., Ste 400, Rockville, MD 20850; (301) 294-5400.

> The most comprehensive source for national health resources and organizations compiled in one book. Profiles of 360 organizations—76 federal agencies and programs, 251 private groups, and 33 foundations (1991). Highlights activities, publications, meetings, and databases.

National AIDS Information Clearinghouse: (800) 458-5231.

A service of the Centers for Disease Control and Prevention, pamphlet called *Understanding AIDS* is available in several languages including Chinese. Health planners will want to order the *Business Responds to AIDS: Manager's Kit*—a variety of self-help materials on planning and implementing a comprehensive workplace HIV/AIDS policy and education program. Call for a publications catalog.

National Cancer Institute, Bldg 31, Room 10A24, Bethesda, MD 20892; (800) 4-CANCER.

Write or call for diet, nutrition, and cancer prevention booklets. One series is designed to be particularly easy to read, and readability levels as low as third grade are indicated. Spanish language brochures are available. Ask about African American booklets such as *Get a New Attitude About Cancer* and Native American brochure *Traditional Foods Can Be Healthy.* All NCI publications are free, but quantities may be limited.

National Center for Health Statistics, Division of Health Promotion Statistics, 6525 Belcrest Road, Hyattsville, MD 20782; (301) 436-7032.

Oversees the collection of national and state data for Healthy People 2000. A reliable source for current information on racial and ethnic populations, including *Healthy People 2000 Review, 1992* (August 1993). See also **Healthy People 2000** and **Office of Disease Prevention and Health Promotion.**

National Center for Nutrition and Dietetics of the American Dietetic Association, 216 W. Jackson Blvd., Chicago, Il 60606-6995; (312) 899-0040; orders (800) 745-0775, ext. 5000.

Comprehensive catalog of publications and services of this membership organization and its collaborative nutrition projects includes the following products of interest to worksite planners and more:

Ethnic and regional food practices—a series of professional manuals or consumer pamphlets to adapt cultural diets and traditional foods. Covers practices, customs, and holiday foods for Alaska Native, Mexican-American, Chinese, Navajo, Hmong, and Jewish populations.

Developing Health Education Materials for Special Audiences: Low-Literate Adults includes an audiotape and study guide. Describes readability and includes guidelines for adapting existing health education materials.

Recipe book for the African American family, *Down Home Healthy* emphasizes low fat and high taste. Written and produced in cooperation with Project LEAN, the National Cancer Institute, and the National Heart, Lung, and Blood Institute.

National Coalition of Hispanic Health & Human Services Organizations, see **COSSMHO.**

National Health Information Center, PO Box 1133, Washington, DC, 20013-1133; (800) 336-4797.

Operated by the Office of Disease Prevention and Health Promotion, an excellent resource for many helpful guides on general health topics and booklets on corporate health promotion published by the federal government. Source for Healthy People 2000 information and updates. Most are free.

National Heart, Lung, and Blood Institute (NHLBI) Information Center, PO Box 30105, Bethesda, MD 20824-0105; (301) 251-1222.

Responds to phone and mail requests related to high blood pressure, cholesterol, smoking, asthma, heart attack, obesity, and blood resources as well as information requests associated with cardiovascular disease prevention and heart health and provides educational materials on these topics (some available in Spanish). Will send up to 10 copies of booklets and publications free; otherwise, postage and handling fees are assessed. Also available are professional materials on heart and lung health in the workplace and free newsletters. Ask for a publications list and to be placed on the mailing list.

Of special interest: *Making Investments for a Healthy Tomorrow,* a free booklet published by the NHLBI Minority Outreach: Research and Education project; and *Strategies for Diffusing Health Information to Minority Populations.*

National Maternal and Child Health Clearinghouse, 8201 Greensboro Drive, Ste 600, McLean, VA 22102; (703) 821-8955, ext. 254.

Distributes current information materials from an inventory of more than 500 titles as part of the government's Maternal and Child Health Bureau. Various booklets and audiovisual information on family planning, prenatal care, newborn care, nutrition, and other family health issues—most are free. Some publications are available in Spanish,

Cambodian, Chinese, Korean, Laotian, Samoan, Tagalog, Thai, and Vietnamese. Call or write for a current publications catalog. Of special interest: *Unity Through Diversity: A Report of the Healthy Mothers, Healthy Babies Coalition; Patient Education Materials: A Resource Guide; Ethnocultural Resource Directory: A Resource Guide for Health Care Professionals Needing Medical Information for the English, Hispanic, and Haitian Client.*

Of particular interest is *Strategies for Working with Culturally Diverse Communities and Clients* by Elizabeth Randall-David (Association for the Care of Children's Health), 1989. Includes a lengthy and thorough discussion of verbal and nonverbal communication systems and family and religious beliefs among various racial and ethnic groups that shape their attitudes toward health (one copy free).

National Medical Association, 1012 Tenth St., NW, Washington, DC 20001; (202) 347-1895.

A professional membership organization of more than 16,000 physicians, promoting the art of medicine to all sectors of the population, with a primary focus on the health issues related to African Americans and medically underserved. Consumer fact sheets are available on AIDS, dietary fat, obesity, and other health areas of concern for African Americans.

National Minority AIDS Council, 300 Eye St., NE, Ste 400, Washington, DC; (202) 544-1076.

Serves as the major national coalition of frontline community and health organizations to address issues of HIV infection because 46 percent of people infected with the virus are members of racial and ethnic groups. This nonprofit organization publishes informative newsletters, holds regional training programs, offers assistance to community organizations, and provides a voice in national policy making. Write or call for membership information. Corporate memberships are encouraged on various levels, including categories for small business, health care providers, and individuals.

National Urban League, 500 East 62nd St., New York, NY 10021; (212) 310-9000.

Health Is Life booklet and posters show diseases from which African Americans and other racial and ethnic groups suffer in greater numbers.

Office for Substance Abuse Prevention (OSAP), U.S. Dept. of Health and Human Services, Public Health Service, Alcohol, Drug Abuse, and Mental Health Administration.

Cultural Competence for Evaluators—A Guide for Alcohol and Other Drug Abuse Prevention Practitioners Working with Ethnic/Racial Communities (1992) is a good general resource.

Office of Disease Prevention and Health Promotion of the Public Health Service, 330 C St., SW, Room 2132, Washington, DC 20201; (202) 205-8180, Attn: Ashley Files, Coordinator, Community-based and Worksite Health Promotion Projects.

Booklet, *Health Promotion Goes to Work: Programs with an Impact,* chronicles key worksite success stories (one copy free). See also **National Health Information Center** and **Healthy People 2000.**

Office of Minority Health Resource Center, U.S. Dept. of Health and Human Services, Public Health Service, Office of Minority Health, PO Box 37337, Washington, DC 20013-7337; (800) 444-6472.

Established by the federal government as a national resource for minority health information in 1987. Main project activities:

(1) Maintains information on health-related resources available at the federal, state, and local levels that target major racial and ethnic populations. Trained information specialists answer requests from consumers and health professionals (Spanish-speaking staff are available).

(2) Maintains a computerized database of health-related publications, organizations, and programs on minority health priority areas and risks. Includes sources of free or low-cost services and materials. New service will help locate funding sources. Customized computer searches are comprehensive and helpful.

(3) The Resource Center will put callers in touch with professionals who are active in a variety of disciplines and who can provide expert technical assistance.

(4) Free publications to ask for:

Closing the Gap. Series of four-page fact sheets that describe the extent to which specific minority groups are affected, present avenues for prevention, and offer other sources of assistance. Selected topics: *Health and Minorities in the U.S.; Chemical Dependency and Minorities; Nutrition;*

> *Diabetes and Minorities; Heart Disease, Stroke, and Minorities; Infant Mortality, Low Birthweight, and Minorities; AIDS/HIV Infection and Minorities.*
>
> *Report of the Secretary's Task Force on Black and Minority Health,* vol. 1, executive summary (available in limited quantity while supplies last), Dept. of Health and Human Services, 1985. The key report in defining the problems; dated in time but not in information.
>
> The following flyers list specific health-related organizations and publications:
>
> *Health Materials for Black Americans*
> *Sources of Health Materials for Asian and Pacific Islander Populations*
> *Sources of Health Materials for Native Americans*
> *Sources of Spanish Language Health Materials*
> *Audiovisual Materials for Minority Populations*

Porter-Novelli, public relations firm, 1120 Connecticut Ave., NW, 11th floor, Washington, DC 20036; (202) 973-5874.

> *Directory of African-American Nutrition Programs*— an extensive guide for identifying organizations and resources published by the National Council of Negro Women and The Procter & Gamble Company— the first project of this partnership called the African-American Nutritional Health Initiative.
>
> *Reweaving the Tapestry of America,* a summary of a conference and vision called "Cross Talk"—a new approach to multicultural communication. Each free.

Program for Appropriate Technology in Health (PATH),
1990 M St., NW, Ste 700, Washington, DC 20036; (202)
822-0033.

> *Developing Health and Family Planning Print
> Materials for Low-Literate Audiences: A Guide*, $5
> prepaid.

The Quaker Oats Company, Consumer Response Dept.,
(312) 222-7843.

> Pamphlets with tips on healthy eating, nutritious
> recipes—some available in Spanish.

Stanford Center for Research in Disease Prevention,
Health Promotion Resource Center, 1000 Welch Road, Palo
Alto, CA 94304-1885; (415) 723-0003.

> Print and video materials developed for use during
> the Stanford Heart Disease Prevention study are now
> available to the general public. Topics cover general
> heart health, nutrition, weight control, smoking,
> blood pressure, exercise, alcohol, and others—many
> items available in Spanish including the *Heart
> Health Test*—a brief assessment and video—and *Por
> la Vida*—a bilingual leader's manual explains this
> program in which Hispanic women learn to lead
> groups of their friends and neighbors to discuss
> nutrition and other family health issues.

> Also, *Restoring Balance: Community-Directed Health
> Promotion for American Indians and Alaska Natives*, a
> manual, provides step-by-step advice for Native
> Americans to improve the health of their own com-
> munities. Examples of how tribes throughout North
> America have met health challenges. Lessons for the
> workplace.

> Worksite planners can learn cultural sensitivity from
> community outreach strategies presented in *Health*

Promotion in Diverse Cultural Communities by Virginia Gonzales and colleagues—a 56-page manual (1991). Useful checklists and many helpful ideas. Call or write for a free catalog of all products.

U.S. Department of Agriculture, Human Nutrition Information Service, Room 346, 6505 Belcrest Road, Hyattsville, MD 20782.

Write for a listing of publications. Of special interest is *Making Healthy Food Choices*—nutrition information for adults with low literacy skills. This 20-page booklet, written at a fifth- to sixth-grade reading level, covers topics such as eating less salt, fat, and cholesterol, shopping for food, and watching weight. Designed for easy reproduction. Order from: Superintendent of Documents, Government Printing Office, Washington, DC 20402 (stock no. 001-000-04592-0; $1.50/each; send check or money order).

Also send for a catalog of other government publications on health through the Consumer Information Center, Pueblo, CO 81009.

EDITOR'S NOTE: WELCOA has attempted to provide accurate details on the organizations and their resources listed here. You may order materials or seek further information directly from the original source. Certainly, some of these addresses and phone numbers may change over time. Prices may vary too. Although we reviewed most of these materials, WELCOA does not specifically endorse any resources or make a judgment on the quality of products described here. And because of the changing nature of health promotion, we cite only materials released in the last few years. WELCOA has tried to be inclusive but not exhaustive, and we admit we may have overlooked some important resources.

ARTICLES

Aguirre-Molina, Marilyn and Carlos W. Molina. Ethnic/racial populations and worksite health promotion. *Occupational Medicine: State of the Art Reviews,* vol. 5, no. 4, October-December 1990, pp. 789-806. Philadelphia, Hanley & Belfus.

Blaisdell, Richard Kekuni. The health status of *Kanaka Maoli* (indigenous Hawaiians). *Asian American and Pacific Islander Journal of Health,* vol. 1., no. 2, autumn 1993, pp. 116-160.

Breslow, Lester, M.D. Empowerment, not outreach: Serving the health promotion needs of the inner city. *American Journal of Health Promotion,* vol. 7, no. 1, September/October 1992, pp. 7-8.

Chen, Moon S., Jr. and colleagues. Lessons learned and baseline data from initiating smoking cessation research with Southeast Asian adults. *Asian American and Pacific Islander Journal of Health,* vol. 1, no. 2, autumn 1993, pp. 194-214.

Health Education, special issue: Health education intervention (health education issues among racial and ethnic minority populations in the United States), December 1989. Publication of the American Alliance for Health, Physical Education, Recreation and Dance.

JAMA: Journal of the American Medical Association. Jan. 9, 1991. Entire issue devoted to Hispanic health issues.

Jamieson, David and Julie O'Mara. *Managing Workforce 2000: Gaining the Diversity Advantage.* San Francisco: Jossey-Bass, 1991.

Jha, Prabhat and colleagues. Coronary artery disease in Asian Indians: Prevalence and risk factors. *Asian American and Pacific Islander Journal of Health*, vol. 1., no. 2, autumn 1993, pp. 161-175.

Lacey, Ella P. U.S. Census procedures: A backdrop for consideration of ethnic and racial issues in health education programming. *Journal of Health Education*, vol. 23, no. 1, January-February 1992, pp. 14-21.

Leslie, Maryann and Carol K. Mikanowicz. The significance of cultural differences and characteristics in program development. *Wellness Perspectives: Research, Theory and Practice*, vol. 9, no. 1, 1992, pp. 24-34.

Lin-Fu, Jane S. Population characteristics and health care needs of Asian Pacific Americans. *Public Health Reports*, vol. 103, no. 1, January-February 1988, pp. 18-27.

Nickens, Herbert W. Health promotion and disease prevention among minorities. *Health Affairs*, summer 1990, pp. 133-143.

Sorlie, Paul D. and colleagues. Mortality by Hispanic status in the United States. *Journal of the American Medical Association*, vol. 270, no. 20, Nov. 24, 1993, pp. 2464-2468.

Sullivan, Louis W. Health promotion and improving access to care for all Americans. *Response* (a publication of the Center for Corporate Public Involvement), November 1990, pp. 15-16.

Thomas, R. Roosevelt, Jr. *Beyond Race and Gender, Unleashing the Power of Your Total Work Force by Managing Diversity*. New York: American Management Assoc., 1991.

APPENDIX

Here is an employee survey to be used as a model for your worksite assessment process. The employee survey presents questions designed to ascertain the nature, level, and types of diversity, and individual and family beliefs, practices, and experiences that may help you better understand your employee groups and plan health promotion programs for them.

You may use these survey questions as a guide as you develop your own instruments and evaluation.

EMPLOYEE SURVEY

Our company is interested in determining the most effective way to work with our employees and improve their health and possibly the health of their families and significant others. Please review and answer the following questions as best you can. We would like to have your name and job title completed only if you feel comfortable in doing so. if not, please check the item (✔ I wish to remain anonymous).

If you have any questions or concerns regarding the collection or use of this information please contact ( ). Personal information gathered will remain confidential. This information will be helpful in developing our company's health promotion program services to better serve you as an individual employee or in helping construct activities for groups of employees with similar. health needs and interests.

Thank you for your help.

Employee Name   Job Title

(_____I wish to remain anonymous)

1. Please describe the city, town, area of the U.S. (or other country) where you and members of your family were born and raised.

2. Did you attend elementary, junior, and senior high school in this same area? If not, please briefly describe where you attended these schools.

3. Do you and/or members of your family speak a language other than English? If so, please indicate which one(s) and if you are able to also write and read in this language as well.

4. What is your earliest memory of visiting the doctor, hospital, or clinic for medical or health care services?

5. Please describe your most significant (positive/negative/both) experience with a medical or health care professional and organization.

6. Have these experiences affected your ideas, attitudes, or belief about medicine and health? In what ways?

7. What does "being healthy" or "feeling well" mean to you?

8. Briefly describe the times in your life when you believe you were the healthiest or feeling the best?

9. Briefly describe the times in your life when you have felt the worst, most ill, or sick.

10. Did your family have any "home remedies" or treatments for the times when you were sick, had a headache, or other health problem? If so, briefly describe what these were and if you still practice some of these remedies.

11. Today, what are the issues that most concern you in your professional life, with your family, or significant others in the community or in our country?

12. What do you believe were the most important things taught to you as you were growing up by family, relatives, or friends?

13. What types of health, education, or recreation programs and activities offered through our company would be of most interest to you? Briefly explain why.

14. Would you want the opportunity to involve your spouse, significant other, children, other family members, or friends as part of these activities? Briefly state why or why not.

15. Would you be interested through our company's health promotion program in sharing with other employees a special skill, ability, or talent you have? If so, what would you like the opportunity to share with them?

16. What talents, skills, or abilities would you enjoy learning from other employees or possibly from volunteers with community organizations?

17. What is the single most important health or medical issue that interests you or you are most concerned about? Briefly describe why you feel this way.

18. What types of things would a health, education, or recreational program have to offer in order for you to regularly participate or attend?

19. Identify one person or group (outside of family members) for whom you have the most respect or admiration and describe why.

20. Please list or describe any other information, advice, concerns, or thoughts you have that may be used to help the health promotion program best serve the needs of all employees in this company.

Notes

Chapter 1

1. *National Survey of Worksite Health Promotion Activities.* Office of Disease Prevention and Health Promotion, 1992.
2. R. Roosevelt Thomas, Jr. *Beyond Race and Gender, Unleashing the Power of Your Total Work Force by Managing Diversity.* New York: American Management Assoc., 1991, pp. 10-11.
3. *Omaha World-Herald,* Associated Press, June 9, 1993.
4. *USA TODAY,* Dec. 4, 1992, p. 8A.
5. David Jamieson and Julie O'Mara. *Managing Workforce 2000: Gaining the Diversity Advantage.* San Francisco: Jossey-Bass, 1991.
6. *Public Health Reports, Journal of the U.S. Public Health Service.* Special Section: Papers from the CDC-ATSDR workshop on the use of race and ethnicity in public health surveillance, vol. 109, no. 1, January-February 1994.
7. Warren, Rueben C. and colleagues. EDITORIAL: The use of race and ethnicity in public health surveillance. *Public Health Reports, Journal of the U.S. Public Health Service.* Special Section: Papers from the CDC-ATSDR workshop on the use of race and ethnicity in public health surveillance, vol. 109, no. 1, January-February 1994, pp. 4-6.
8. Marilyn Aguirre-Molina and Carlos W. Molina. Ethnic/racial populations and worksite health promotion, in *Occupational Medicine: State of the Art Reviews,* vol. 5, no. 4, October-December 1990, pp. 789-806.

Chapter 2

1. Howard N. Fullerton. The American work force, 1992-2005: Another look at the labor force. *Monthly Labor Review,* November 1993, pp. 31-40.
2. Michael A. Stoto, Ruth Behrens, and Connie Rosemont (editors). *Healthy People 2000: Citizens Chart the Course.* Washington, D.C.: National Academy Press, 1990.
3. Testimony at the Healthy People 2000 hearings was reported in *Healthy People 2000: Citizens Chart the Course.* Text is excerpted, paraphrased, and summarized here with written permission from the National Academy Press, Washington, D.C.

4. Testimony from John Waller, Wayne State University, in *Healthy People 2000: Citizens Chart the Course.*
5. Moon S. Chen, Jr., and colleagues. Lessons learned and baseline data from initiating smoking cessation research with Southeast Asian adults. *Asian American and Pacific Islander Journal of Health,* vol. 1, no. 2, autumn 1993, pp. 194-214.
6. T. Guillermo. Testimony before the U.S. House of Representatives, Jan. 24, 1994. Tessie Guillermo is Executive Director of the Asian American Health Forum in San Francisco.
7. Office of Disease Prevention and Health Promotion, 1993.
8. *USA TODAY,* April 15, 1991.
9. National Center for Health Statistics. *Health, United States, 1991* and *Prevention Profile.*
10. *INFOMEMO,* National Heart, Lung and Blood Institute, July 1991, p. 14. See also, Richard Kekuni Blaisdell, The health status of Kanaka Maoli (indigenous Hawaiians). *Asian American and Pacific Islander Journal of Health,* vol. 1, no. 2, autumn 1993, pp. 116-160.
11. Chen and colleagues, 1993.
12. Jenkins and colleagues. Cancer risks among Vietnamese refugees, *Western Journal of Medicine,* vol. 5, no. 1, 1990, pp. 15-20.
13. Blaisdell, 1993.
14. Prabhat Jha and colleagues. Coronary artery disease in Asian Indians: Prevalence and risk factors. *Asian American and Pacific Islander Journal of Health,* vol. 1, no. 2, autumn 1993, pp. 161-175.
15. Indian Health Service, 1993.
16. *INFOMEMO, NHLBI,* February 1991, p. 15.
17. *American Journal of Health Promotion.*

Chapter 3

1. *Strategies for Diffusing Health Information to Minority Populations.* National Heart, Lung and Blood Institute, 1987.

Chapter 4

1. *Network News,* Asian American Health Forum, spring 1992.
2. Adapted from information supplied by David M. Hunnicutt, PhD, and Margaret A. Mann, Alcoholism and Drug Abuse Council of Nebraska; and Joe Leutzinger, PhD, Union Pacific Railroad.
3. *JAMA: Journal of the American Medical Association,* Jan. 9, 1991.

Chapter 5

1. *Developing Health and Family Planning Print Materials for Low-Literate Audiences: A Guide.* Program for Appropriate Technology in Health (PATH), p. 48, fig. 31, used with permission.

About the Author

Stephen Ramirez, MPH, is division manager of Health Promotion Services with the Fresno County Health Services Agency in California. In this capacity he administers an operating budget well over $1 million and supervises 14 professional staff engaged in disease prevention and health promotion activities for a large, racially and ethnically diverse metropolitan/rural community.

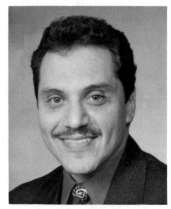

Stephen Ramirez

Steve has worked in both the public and private sectors. His 15 years of professional and consulting assignments in the health and human services field have enabled Steve to train professionals and community leaders in the delivery of health promotion programs reaching diverse populations across the United States.

Some of his accomplishments include providing prevention programs to high-risk youth and families in the areas of substance abuse, violence, adolescent pregnancy, child safety, and the design of a comprehensive community plan for the prevention and control of tobacco use.

His national child safety and survival program received special recognition from a Presidential Commission. He helped develop a public affairs series devoted to community health issues with a local NBC-TV affiliate in California. And he has organized and produced health education videos on tuberculosis and AIDS in two languages, English and Spanish. Steve also developed guidelines for practicing health education and health promotion in a managed care system.

Steve's work with local, state, and national organizations also includes the development and delivery of training to health education professionals, board members, and community leaders in all regions of the United States. He has presented sessions at over 20 different national, state, and regional conferences primarily on the topic of providing health promotion and wellness programs to diverse populations and the medically underserved.

He is a member of the National Wellness Institute's Board of Trustees and also has been the Multi-Cultural Education Track Chairperson for the Association for Worksite Health Promotion annual conferences (1992 and 1993).

A native New Yorker, Steve was born and raised in the Bronx and earned a bachelor's degree in health education from Hunter College and a master's degree in public health from Columbia University.

About Wellness Councils of America

The Wellness Councils of America—known widely as WELCOA—is a national nonprofit organization dedicated to promoting healthier lifestyles for all Americans, especially through health promotion activities at the worksite.

WELCOA has a nationwide network of locally affiliated Wellness Councils serving corporate members and their employees. At the same time, WELCOA acts as a national clearinghouse and information center on corporate health promotion for companies everywhere.

This book is just one example of the types of products WELCOA develops and distributes on corporate health promotion. Other products include manuals, videos, and brochures—most notably, WELCOA's premier resource *Healthy, Wealthy & Wise: Fundamentals of Workplace Health Promotion*, now in its third edition.

Working Together

WELCOA came into being in 1985 as a "Wellness Councils of America" project of the Health Insurance Association of America. Two years later, WELCOA was launched as a nonprofit Nebraska corporation with headquarters in Omaha.

The seeds of WELCOA, however, were planted in 1982 when Omaha employers joined together to form the nation's first Wellness Council. Its mission was, and is, to enhance the health and well-being of employees to improve productivity, reduce absenteeism, and contain escalating health care costs. The Omaha Council's success spurred cost-conscious employers in other communities to form their own Wellness Councils under WELCOA's umbrella.

Building Healthy Workplaces

WELCOA has launched a nationwide program called WELL CITY USA and its work-site component, Well Workplace. The Well City project originated with the Wellness Council of the Midlands in Columbia, South Carolina. In 1991, WELCOA adapted WELL CITY USA for its membership and tested the project through its network.

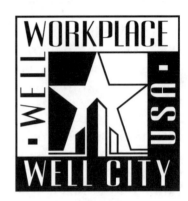

WELCOA, drawing on years of experience in health promotion and testing the concepts through its national network, developed Well Workplace to address two fundamental questions:

"How do we get health promotion started or what do we do next?

and

"What makes a worksite health promotion program successful?"

Well Workplace establishes criteria to measure the success of corporate health promotion—as a model for companies to use in forming their own programs—and rewards companies who achieve Well Workplace objectives. Companies who meet the objectives join WELCOA's roster of "America's Healthiest Companies."

Until now, there has been no standard for what health promotion should be and how it fits into the corporate quality management and cost-containment structure. Well Workplace allows this integration—a blending of the components that are required to improve employee health status and to contain health care costs.

Change through leadership is accomplished by WELCOA's prestigious board of directors, strategically positioned to deal with national health-related issues, including health care reform issues. WELCOA has joined an alliance of organizations whose purpose is to ensure that reform proposals contain incentives for employers to carry out worksite health promotion programs.

For complete information about the Wellness Councils of America, including a publications list and membership information, call or write

Wellness Councils of America
Community Health Plaza, Suite 311
7101 Newport Ave.
Omaha, NE 68152
(402) 572-3590

Index

mission statement , developing, 14-16
    for health promotion program, 14
National AIDS Information Clearinghouse
    resource information, 118
National Cancer Institute, resource information, 118
National Center for Health Statistics
    resource information, 118
National Center for Nutrition and Dietetics
    resource information, 119
National Coalition of Hispanic Health & Human Services
    Organizations, see COSSMHO
National Health Information Center
    resource information, 119-120
National Heart, Lung, and Blood Institute, resource information, 120
National Maternal and Child Health Clearinghouse
    resource information, 120-121
National Medical Association, resource information, 121
National Minority AIDS Council
    resource information, 121-122
National Urban League, resource information, 122
Native Americans, 37
    health profile, 45-47
    health status, 27-49
    labor force participation, 28
    organizations, 110, see also Indian Health Service
    resources, 125
    risks, 41
Native Hawaiians, 43, see also Asian and Pacific Islander Americans
needs assessment, 59-64, sample survey, 129-132
nutrition, program ideas, 77-80
    resources, 109, 114, 117, 119, 124, 125, 126
obesity, 35, 43, 45
occupational safety, program ideas, 88
Office for Substance Abuse Prevention, resource information, 122
Office of Disease Prevention and Health Promotion
    resource information, 122
Office of Minority Health Resource Center
    resource information, 123-124
organ donation, 93
Pacific Gas & Electric, 5
physical activity and fitness, program ideas, 81-83
Porter-Novelli, resource information, 124
poverty, 32-33, 39, 46
prenatal care, prenatal programs, 40, 45
    Marriott, 10
    resources, 116
    see also maternal and infant health and infant mortality